Workouts
for Women

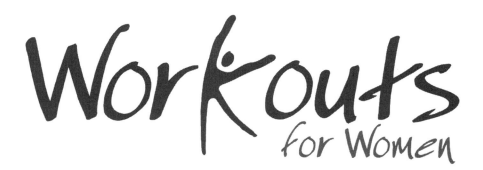

Workouts for Women

WEIGHT TRAINING

Joni Hyde

Photographs by Peter Field Peck

healthyliving**books**
New York • London

A HEALTHY LIVING BOOK
Published by
Hatherleigh Press
5-22 46th Avenue, Suite 200
Long Island City, NY 11101
www.healthylivingbooks.com

  ISBN-13: 978-1-57826-210-6
  ISBN-10: 1-57826-210-0

Library of Congress Cataloging-in-Publication Data

Hyde, Joni.
  Workouts for women : weight training / Joni Hyde.
      p. cm.
  ISBN 1-57826-210-0
  1. Weight training for women. 2. Excercise for women. I. Title.
  GV546.6.W64H93 2005
  613.7'045--dc22
                                            2005028089

Seek the advice of your physician before starting any physical fitness program.

Healthy Living Books are available for bulk purchase, special promotions, and premiums.
For information on reselling and special purchase opportunities, please call us at 1-800-
528-2550 and ask for the Special Sales Manager.

Cover and interior design by Deborah Miller.

10 9 8 7 6 5 4 3 2 1
Printed in Canada

Table of Contents

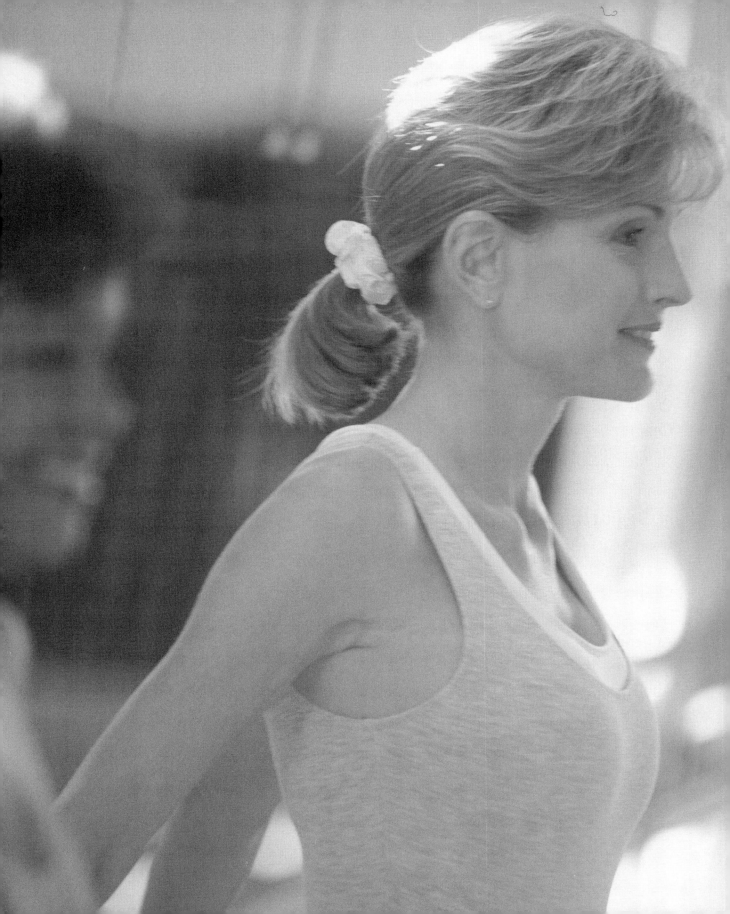

Introduction

Welcome Back to

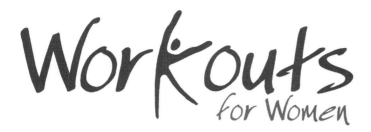

Welcome to *Workouts for Women: Weight Training*! For those of you currently using the *Workouts for Women: Circuit Shaping* book, *Workouts for Women: Weight Training* will perfectly complement your exercise regimen. This book will help you tailor your fitness program to the unique needs you may encounter as you focus on sculpting your body. Even if you are new to the Workouts for Women approach to fitness, we are confident that you will immediately feel inspired to begin our easy-to-follow weight training exercises.

I understand that women sometimes get lost in the juggle of family, work, home and community obligations. Our personal indulgences and self-improvement often remain last and sometimes don't even make the list! Because of these special obstacles women face, I have created a flexible weight training program that can be contoured to fit your particular needs and time constraints. Exercises are grouped into short 15 Minute Zone Workouts which allow you to target specific areas of the body. You plan out your fitness program and work out in the comfort of your own home!

Exercise is critical for effective weight control and positive lifestyle maintenance, providing both physical and mental benefits. Because of media oversaturation, we may tune out the importance of this concept. Weight training will improve the way you perceive your body and boost your self-esteem. Beyond body image, weight training ultimately provides health benefits, such as decreased risk for osteoporosis, increased muscle strength, increased flexibility and movement, developed coordination and balance. All of these contribute to an improved quality of life.

Get ready to continue (or start!) down the path toward a better, healthier and happier you. It all begins with exercise, so take that step toward a more empowered you!

Stay fit and healthy.

Joni Hyde

Joni Hyde, Your Personal Trainer

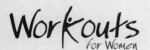

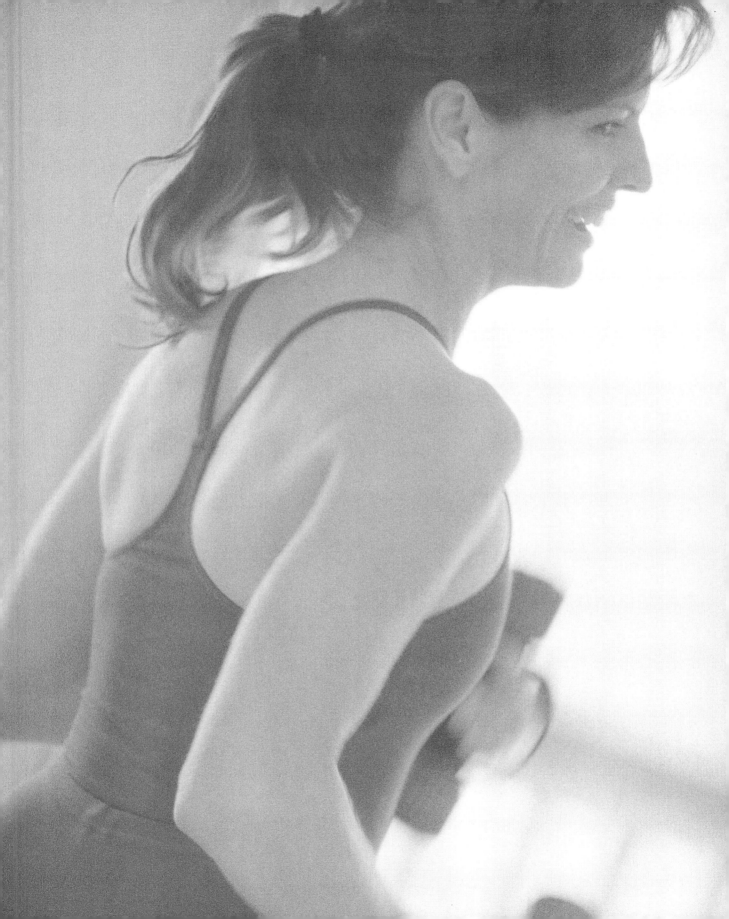

Part

1

Weight Training
Is For Women, Too!

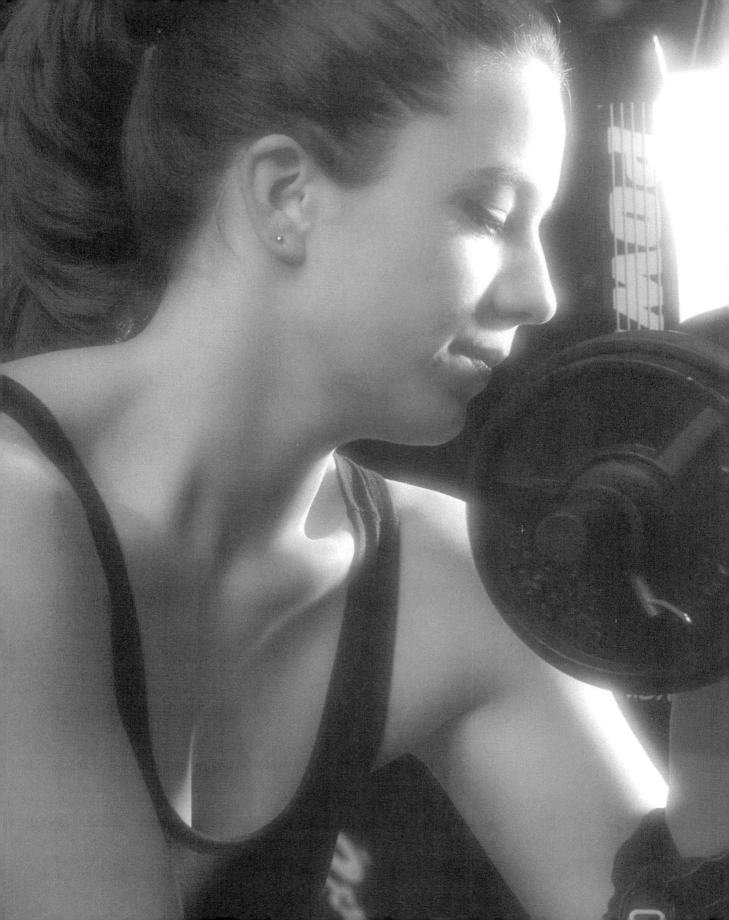

CHAPTER 1

Weight Training Unveiled

Dispel The Weight Training Myths

Do you only associate weight training with a room full of men, muscles bulging as they exert all their strength upon heavy weights? Prepare to become enlightened as you enter the Workouts for Women world of weight training. Many women have experienced positive effects and health benefits from weight training and so can you.

One myth is that weight training will cause women to develop a masculine physique. However, a woman's body responds differently to weight training than a man's body due to hormonal properties. Testosterone is the hormone which causes men to build up muscles more dramatically than women. Every woman is an individual and comprises certain genetic characteristics. This will affect the development of your own unique shape in response to weight training.

Women are plagued by entirely different physical issues than men. Our primary concern is body shape and body composition. We want to be firm and lean. We want delicate feminine muscle tone and sculpted hips, thighs, buttocks and arms. In many cases, women want to not only firm up problem areas, but often to reduce the size of these areas. Aerobic exercise produces numerous benefits and cannot be replaced. However, aerobic exercise does not tone muscle, and muscle tone is key to a well-sculpted body. In order to achieve the best body shape possible, you must incorporate weight training into your fitness routines.

In addition to the visible physical changes, weight training positively affects your health. Some of the rewards are increased bone density, increased metabolism, increased strength, increased muscle mass and decreased body mass. All these have an impact on the prevention of various health afflictions. With consistency, weight training will give you the physique you desire while reversing some of the inevitable results of aging. Be prepared for some welcome changes as you begin your Workouts for Women weight training program.

What Is Weight Training?

Weight training is a type of exercise in which your body works against the force of gravity. Weight training utilizes the Overload Principle which states that muscle size, strength and endurance will only improve when the resistance encountered is greater than what you are used to.

Weight training is progressive, which means that as you become stronger, the weight lifted must be increased proportionally if further gains are desired. In order to avoid plateaus, you may need to reassess and alter your program periodically. Some of the changes could be an increase in the amount of weight lifted, an increase in the number of sets worked, completely changing the actual exercises or even a modification of the rest intervals between sets.

Weight training is specific. Simply put, the development of muscular fitness is directly related to the muscles trained. Weight training can be focused on particular targeted areas of your body.

Weight Training Works!

If you want to see visible results fast, nothing compares with using weights to tone your body and burn excess fat while simultaneously decreasing various health risks, decreasing your risk for injury and enhancing your life overall.

If weight loss is your goal, do not be discouraged by the scale as you begin your program. Because muscle is more dense than fat, you will look and feel healthier before these changes are reflected on the bathroom scale. Focus your attention on the way your clothes look and feel as you add muscle tissue and erase unwanted fat.

One encouraging fact is that you may be pleasantly surprised by the initial rapid results, including a noticeable increase in muscle tone as well as increased strength. However, a strength plateau often occurs several months into a new routine when these initial gains begin to level. This will be your cue that the time has come to increase the challenge since your body is adapting to the workload. When you reach this plateau, do not be discouraged. It is simply a sign that it is time to push yourself to the next level.

Your Metabolism Is Slowing... It's Not Your Imagination!

If you have not experienced it yet, you have certainly heard other women talk about a slowing metabolism that occurs with age. With that slow down comes weight gain even if your eating habits have not changed. The good news is that there is a way to reverse these effects without excessive hours of aerobic activity

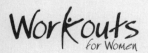

or the newest fad diet. Aerobic activity does nothing to replace or help to maintain muscle mass and fad diets alone will only cause you to lose more muscle mass.

To speed up your metabolism to its original capacity you have to replace the muscle mass that you have lost. The only way to do that is with weight training. Increase your metabolism, shape, tone and shave inches through weight training and defy the odds!

CHAPTER 1
Weight Training Unveiled

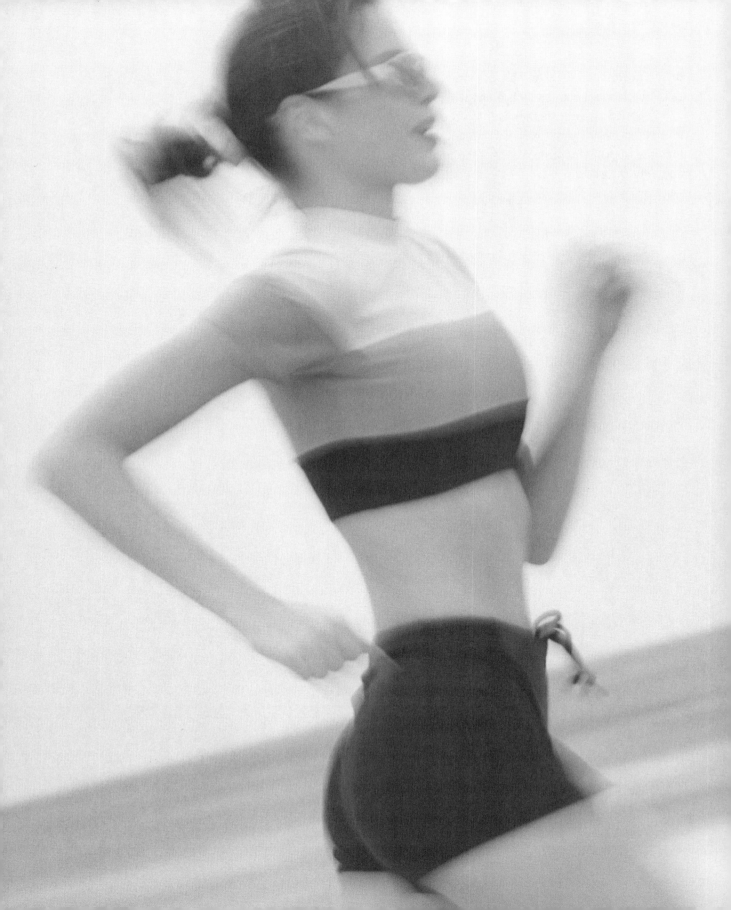

CHAPTER 2

Planning Your Workouts

Set Your Sights

If you fail to plan, then you plan to fail. The first step in developing your weight training program is to decide what you want to accomplish and commit to your personal objectives. Only you can choose to believe in yourself and your ability to be consistent, stay focused on your goals and persevere. Much can be accomplished with a positive mindset. Your outer strength is reliant on your inner strength. Be sure to channel goal-setting energy toward personally stimulating and motivating forces, rather than detached goals that someone else has set for you.

Weight training is beneficial for the physical and emotional health of all generations and no matter what age you are, you are never too old to begin. At any age you are empowering your body with strength, providing the ability to recover more quickly after injury or illness and investing time in developing good healthy lifetime habits that can bring forth great satisfaction. Fitness is not just a short term activity, but a permanent plan to incorporate into your life.

Finding the time to exercise can be tough, but if you make a plan and schedule your workout time in advance, you will be much more likely to get it done. With kids, jobs, school and all the other responsibilities of home and family, where does exercise fit in? First, make exercise a priority. If you are serious about getting fit, you will find time to exercise. Begin by writing down your typical schedule and block out time for exercise. Work out at the same time every day. If you make it a daily routine, it becomes your special time to take care of yourself.

Once you start, you will quickly recognize the sense of vitality that comes with your newfound strength. Plan to continually learn more about health and fitness for your own well-being and share your knowledge with others. Take pleasure in learning the proper form so that your weight training sessions are as safe and effective as they can be. Above all, do not be in a hurry to accomplish what should be goals to last a lifetime.

As you embark on this journey, keep a positive attitude, refrain from obsessing about missed workouts, do not worry about the last remaining pounds that hang on and especially do not compare your progress to others. Rather, focus on the advances you are making and appreciate that despite the inevitable process of aging, you will be the best YOU that you can be at any age. Enjoy each workout and be grateful for the ability to get up each morning and make it happen!

How Often Can I Weight Train?

ZONE TRAINING CONCEPT

Zone training focuses on manipulating and fatiguing certain areas of your body, in particular the areas you have targeted. This allows substantial flexibility for how you contour the program. For instance, if you specifically want to work on your lower body and abdominals, you would choose the Lower Body Zone workout and the Abdominal Zone workout. Consequently, you would be focusing your entire 30 minutes of weight training on the areas you have selected. The workouts are broken down into the following Zones:

- Shoulders and Arms

- Chest and Back

- Lower Body

- Abdominals and Lower Back

- Total Body

SETS AND REPETITIONS

A few words you will hear repeated time and again are sets and repetitions. It is important that you are aware of what these terms mean so that you will clearly understand the program recommendations. A repetition is one complete full range-of-motion exercise. A set is a group of repetitions. For example, doing three sets of 8 to 12 repetitions of squats means that you will do 8 to 12 squats and then rest. Then you will do 8 to 12 more squats and rest again. Then repeat 8 to 12 squats once more. Your rest periods between sets should be 15 to 30 seconds. Use this time to have a mouthful of water, to stretch and to practice proper breathing.

CYCLING WORKOUTS FOR MAXIMUM RESULTS

Repeating the same style workout over and over causes your body to adapt to this familiar repeated stress. Once your body becomes fully adapted, results will plateau. In order to continue obtaining results over the extended course of time, it is impor-

WHAT TIME IS IT?

Any time is the right time to exercise!

Early Morning Benefits:
* No interruptions or distractions...yet.
* Surveys report more exercise regimen consistency.
* Research indicates a sharper mind for 4 – 10 hours post exercise.
* The energy boost really gets you going.
* Morning exercise helps regulate daily appetite.

Afternoon/Evening Benefits:
* Contrary to previous research, exercise helps you fall asleep faster.
* You are at peak performance.
* Muscles are already warmed up and flexible.
* Exercise is a great stress release.
* Muscles are stronger as the day progresses.

So, pick the best exercise time for you and reap the benefits!

tant to introduce different training techniques into your routine from time to time. Variety is an important factor in the success of your weight training program.

One of the most productive and time-efficient ways to get that variety is by "cycling" your workouts. Cycling is a training method that incorporates systematic change so that you will constantly be training muscles differently. Consequently, your body will not have a chance to get used to one type of workout, which results in plateau. This change could be in the number of repetitions and weight used for a given muscle. It could be a change in the exercise patterns performed or it could be a change in the actual exercises that you complete. Schedules and suggested training patterns that will help you cycle your workouts are offered in Chapter 10.

SCHEDULING

It is a common misconception that an individual should never weight train on back-to-back days. However, depending on a weight lifter's program and goals, it may apply to space out workouts. For instance, weight lifters who have a goal to build mass lift very heavy weight. They train certain body parts only one or two times a week with lots of rest time in between to allow muscles to enlarge at a faster rate. Since this is not a mass-building type of program, we do not have to stick to that rule. For many women, weight training three times a week is adequate to maintain muscle tone. However, if you are just starting out and setting your sights on significantly changing the look of your body quickly, you can weight train up to 5 days a week with two rest days. The key is to not weight train heavily on all 5 days.

PLANNING THE WORKOUT FOR YOUR FITNESS LEVEL

There are 10 different workouts included in this book. Each workout is appropriate for either a beginner, intermediate or advanced exerciser. To increase or decrease the difficulty of your workout, simply increase or decrease the amount of weight you are using. Always choose a weight that allows you to work in the range of 8 to 12 repetitions per each set.

Expect Results And Support Your Goals

Setting up an environment that encourages your success is essential. Talk about your plans and goals with your spouse, family or friends and ask them to gently remind you of your commitments if they see you getting off track. Refuse to let excuses get in the way of your progress and consistency. Life has a way of disrupting well-intentioned plans from time to time, but never make exercise an all or nothing experience. Allow flexibility to come into your plan and mentally prepare for the fact that at times you may miss workouts, possibly days or even weeks, but this is no reason to quit. Get back to your plan and do not agonize over faltering steps.

Progress does not just happen. It takes planning, perseverance and consistency. Visualize a realistic picture of how you want to look and feel. This image will give you direction and the benefits will flow once you decide exactly what you want and begin working toward your goals.

Ninety percent of the women who succeed at reaching and maintaining their fitness goals and living a healthy lifestyle have one major factor in common: They set goals for themselves and write them down. Your goals should be very specific. They should be measurable, attainable and realistic. Have you thought about what your goals are? If not, write them down and map out a timeline of when you want to meet your goals, with checkpoints for rewards along the way. Rewards are great incentives. Give yourself a treat for making all your workout appointments for the week: Manicures and pedicures, a massage and a long bubble bath are all great treats.

If you are trying to lose weight, be realistic and aim to lose 1 to 2 pounds per week. Weight loss that exceeds 2 pounds per week is not healthy and can slow down your metabolism and put you at risk of losing vital muscle tissue. But don't be ruled by the scale. Since muscle weighs more than fat, as you get fit, the numbers on the scale may lead you to think you are not truly losing. In addition to the

INJURY RESPONSE

Even with the most careful execution, injuries can occur during exercise. The most common injuries are related to tendons and ligaments. An important injury regimen every exerciser should know is RICE:

REST – Do not use an injured knee, ankle, shoulder, etc. Rest promotes healing.

ICE – Apply ice to a new injury as soon as possible for about 30 minutes. Cold shrinks torn blood vessels and helps to stop internal bleeding. Re-apply the ice three to five times. Approximately 72 hours after an injury, apply heat periodically if needed for comfort.

COMPRESSION – Wrap the injury firmly, but not too tightly. This will keep swelling down and reduce motion on the injury.

ELEVATION – Raise the injured area above heart level if possible. Gravity drains fluid, which will minimize swelling and pain.

If pain persists for more than 2 or 3 days, you should consult with your health care provider. Also, seek immediate care if there is any loss of joint motion, swelling or sharp or severe pain.

scale, track your progress by the way you feel, with a measuring tape and by the fit of your clothes. A good rule of thumb is to decrease one dress size per month.

As you become stronger, you will find that the accomplishment of a healthier physical self will help to balance other parts of your life as well. Your energy level will be higher, therefore you will have more energy for work and recreation. Your self-esteem will grow and consequently you will feel more empowered and have the confidence to share your new positive energy with others.

Give high priority to time allocated for your weight training program. Prioritize and set aside time especially for YOU several times a week.

Get Ready...Get Set...

Women of all ages are enjoying incredible benefits from lifting weights. Studies have shown that women who lift weights have a reduced risk for osteoporosis while increasing lean muscle mass. This increase in muscle mass maximizes the body's ability to burn calories—even at rest! From the young woman trying to contour her body to the mature woman whose goal is to stay strong, vibrant and healthy, weight lifting is good for everyone. More women realize that proper weight training will produce a leaner, healthier, stronger body without bulky muscles and are incorporating weight training into their overall workout routines. The results are sensational!

Get Fit Now!

Before you begin your workout, be prepared. Fill up your water bottle, put on your favorite music and set up all of your equipment so you can move quickly from one exercise to the next. The time it takes to put on your ankle weights, have a drink of water or get into position for the next exercise is all the rest you should give yourself until you are finished. (However, if you experience any warning signs, such as dizziness, shortness of breath, etc., stop immediately and consult your physician for exercise parameters.) With everything in place, it is time to get moving and there is no better time to shape up. Empower yourself as a woman and make fitness a part of your lifestyle!

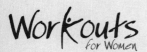

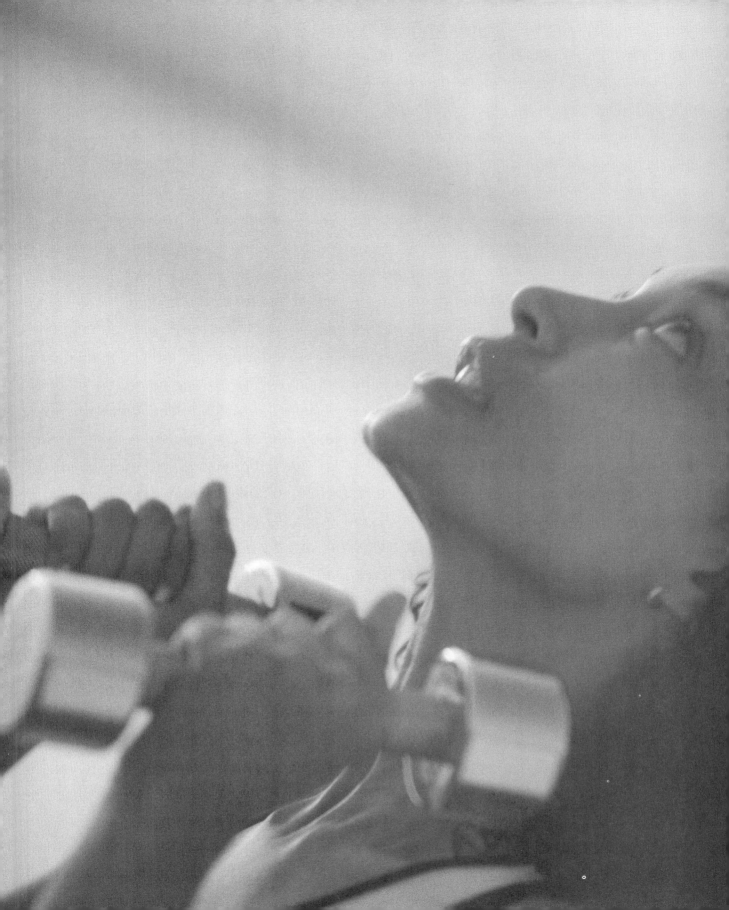

Part
2

Strength Training Exercises

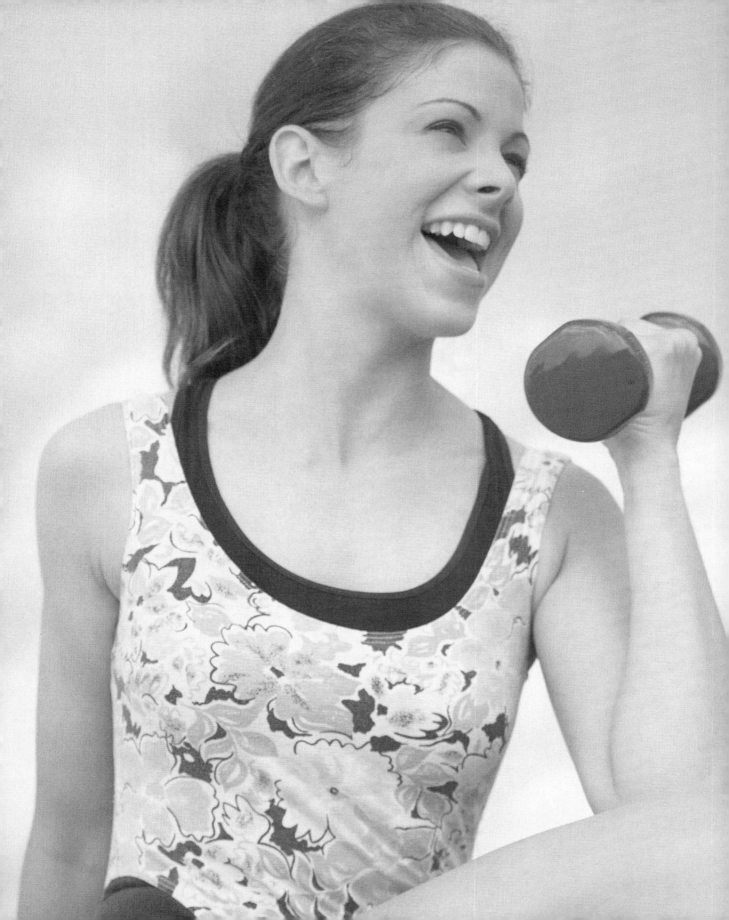

CHAPTER 3

Shoulders and Arms

Shoulders and arms not only are attached, but work as a team. Consequently, they are the joint focal point of one Zone. The muscles in this Zone are a complex pulley system performing magnificent feats. Shoulders and arms have obvious necessary functions, such as lift, carry, push, pull and swing. The front of the arms (biceps) and the back of the arms (triceps) are opposing muscle groups, so exercising them in the same workout creates balance. The triceps can be a particularly difficult spot for women to maintain. Quite frankly though, it is worth the dedication because tightly toned arms and shoulders look great on a woman. Create a fabulous upper body as you trim, sculpt and strengthen. This Zone Workout gives you the tools to channel your energy toward the shoulders as well as the front and back of the upper arms.

ROUTINE A

BODY PART WORKED
Shoulders (Medial Deltoid)

SET UP
Stand tall with legs about shoulder width apart. Grip the bar with hands just outside shoulder width with palms facing toward you. Hold abdominal muscles in tight, shoulders back and chest high.

TIPS FROM JONI
Keep the bar close to your body throughout the move. Keep your shoulders down throughout the move.

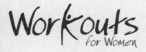

Upright Row With Bar

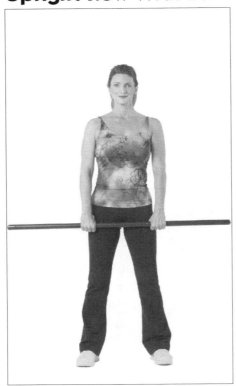 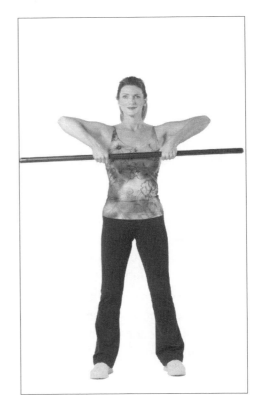

Exercise Technique
1. Bend your elbows up and out to the sides pulling the bar upward, stopping when elbows are shoulder level.

2. Reverse the move and extend your arms back down to start position.

REPEAT 8 TO 12 TIMES.

Overhead Triceps Extension With Bar

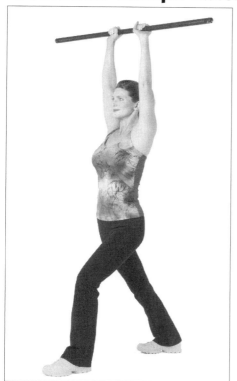 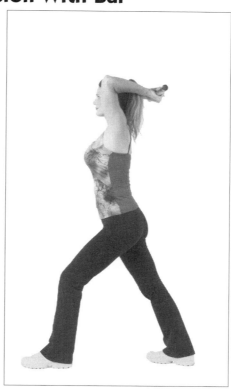

BODY PART WORKED

Back of Arms (Triceps)

SET UP

Stand tall with one leg forward about a foot in front of the other leg and shoulder width apart. Hold abdominal muscles tight, shoulders back and chest high. Grip the bar with hands shoulder width apart with palms facing toward you. Bend your arms at your elbows as you lift the bar over your head with your elbows close to your ears. This is your starting position.

TIPS FROM JONI

Be sure your elbows do not drift, keeping them close to your ears and stationary.

Exercise Technique

1. Bend at the elbows as you lower the bar toward the back of your neck.

2. Exhale as you press the bar straight up to start position, feeling the tension in the back of the arms.

REPEAT 8 TO 12 TIMES.

CHAPTER 3
Shoulders and Arms

ROUTINE A

BODY PART WORKED
Shoulders (Deltoid)

SET UP
Stand tall with one leg forward about a foot in front of the other leg and shoulder width apart. Hold abdominal muscles in tight, shoulders back and chest high. Grip the bar with hands shoulder width apart with palms facing toward you. Bend your arms at your elbows as you lift the bar up to start position, with the bar about chin level. Elbows should be pulled in toward your hips.

TIPS FROM JONI
When extending arms overhead be sure not to overextend by keeping elbows soft. Keep elbows pulled in toward the hips throughout the movement.

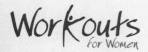

Overhead Bar Press

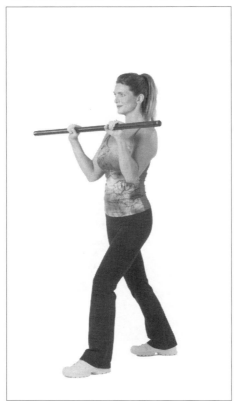 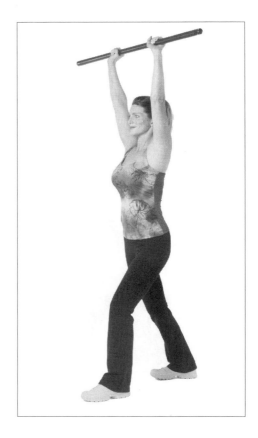

Exercise Technique
1. Exhale as you extend your arms straight up.

2. Lower your arms down to start position, returning the bar to chin height.

REPEAT 8 TO 12 TIMES.

Biceps Curl With Bar

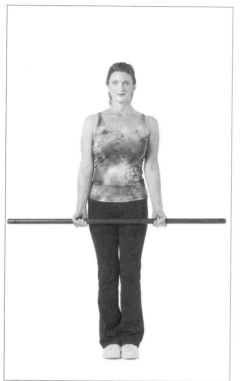 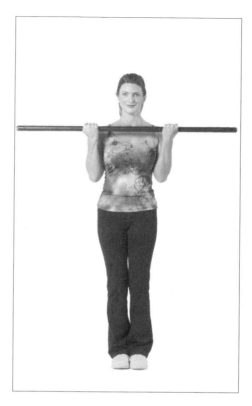

BODY PART WORKED
Front of Arms (Biceps)

SET UP
Stand tall with your shoulders back, chest out and abdominal muscles held in tight. Hold a weighted bar with palms facing out and elbows close at your sides.

TIPS FROM JONI
Be sure not to lock your elbows when lowering your arm back down to start. Keep elbows stationary throughout the move.

Exercise Technique

1. Exhale as you bend your arms at the elbow, bringing the bar up toward your shoulder with palms facing in at the top of the move.

2. Extend your arms back down to start in a controlled manner.

REPEAT 8 TO 12 TIMES.

CHAPTER 3
Shoulders and Arms

ROUTINE A

BODY PART WORKED

Back Of Arms (Triceps)

SET UP

Grip a weighted bar with palms facing toward you and sit down on the floor or the edge of a step. Lie down on the floor or step with head and neck supported and feet flat. Now extend your arms straight up so that the bar is above you with your hands directly above your shoulders.

TIPS FROM JONI

Keeping upper arms motionless with elbows pulled in toward your body on both the lifting and lowering phases is critical to making this exercise effective. If your arms drift forward or backward the focus will not remain on the back of the arms as intended.

Keep your back flat throughout the move. To prevent your back from arching, concentrate on keeping your pelvis slightly lifted.

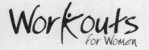

Lying Triceps Extension With Bar

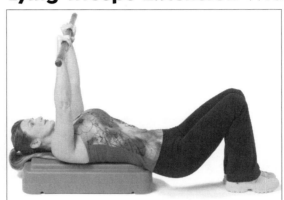

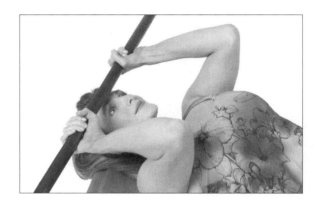

Exercise Technique

1. Keep upper arms motionless and elbows pulled in toward your body as you bend at the elbows, lowering the bar back down in an arc toward your forehead, stopping just before the bar touches you.

2. Exhale and extend your arms, lifting the bar back up to start, feeling the tension in the back of your arms.

REPEAT 8 TO 12 TIMES.

Forward Raise With Bar

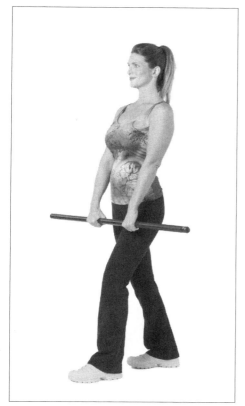 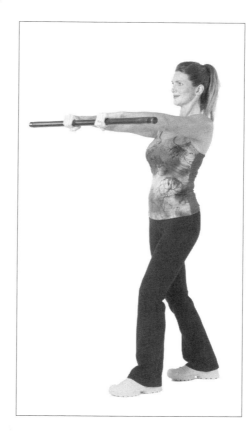

BODY PART WORKED
Front of Shoulders (Medial Deltoid)

SET UP
Stand tall with one leg forward about a foot in front of the other leg and shoulder width apart. Hold abdominal muscles in tight, shoulders back and chest high. Grip the bar in your hands with your palms facing in, resting on your thighs.

TIPS FROM JONI
Keep a slight bend in your knees during this move to release some pressure from your back as you lift the weight up in front of your body.

Exercise Technique
1. Exhale as you raise up the bar directly in front of your body, stopping at shoulder height.

2. Lower the bar back down in a controlled manner.

REPEAT 8 TO 12 TIMES.

CHAPTER 3
Shoulders and Arms

ROUTINE B

BODY PART WORKED

Front of Arms (Biceps)

SET UP

Stand tall with shoulders back, chest high and abdominal muscles held in tight. Hold dumbbells in each hand and stand with feet about shoulder width apart. Place your arms down at your sides with the palms facing in.

TIPS FROM JONI

Keep elbows stationary at your sides throughout the move, being sure they do not move forward or backward.

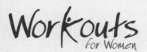

Hammer Curls

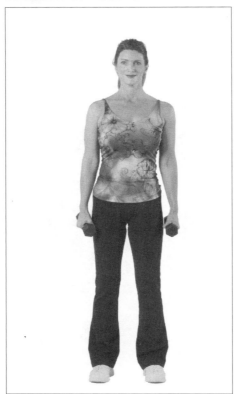 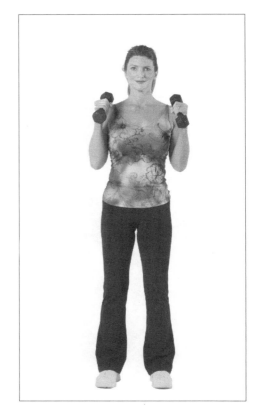

Exercise Technique

1. Exhale as you bend your arms at the elbows, lifting hands up toward your shoulders.

2. Extend arms back down to your sides in a controlled manner.

REPEAT 8 TO 12 TIMES.

Straight Arm Laterals

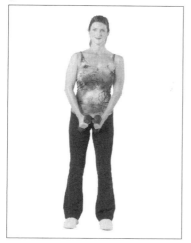
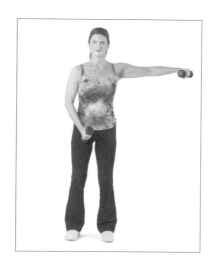
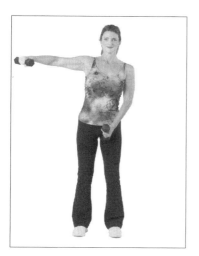
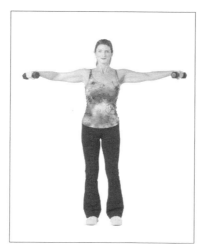

BODY PART WORKED

Sides of Shoulders (Medial Deltoid)

SET UP

Stand tall with feet together and knees slightly bent with shoulders back, chest high and abdominal muscles held in tight. Hold dumbbells in each hand with arms hanging down in front of your body with palms facing toward each other.

TIPS FROM JONI

At the top of the move check for proper form, being sure that hand and elbow are at the same height and that wrist is straight.

Exercise Technique

1. Keep arms straight and exhale as you extend one arm directly out to the side, stopping at shoulder height.

2. Control the resistance as you lower your arm back down to start position.

REPEAT 8 TO 12 TIMES, ALTERNATING ON EACH SIDE.

CHAPTER 3
Shoulders and Arms

ROUTINE B

BODY PART WORKED

Back of Upper Arm (Tricep)

SET UP

Begin this exercise in a semi-lunge position, standing with one leg forward and one back. Both knees should be pointing straight ahead and abdominal muscles should be held in tight. Lean forward, bending at the hip, and rest the forward hand on your forward thigh to support your body. Hold a dumbbell in the other hand and raise the arm up, bending at the elbow so that the upper arm is in line with your torso and close to your body.

TIPS FROM JONI

Keep your elbow stationary and close to your body throughout the move. Be sure not to swing the working arm. Concentrate on using the muscles in the back of your arm to lift the weight.

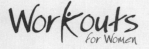

Bent Over Tricep Kickback

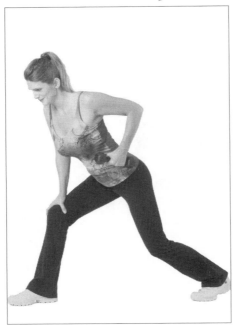 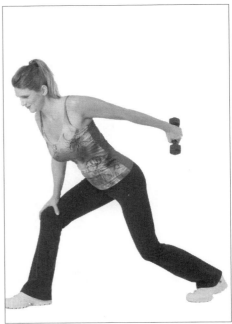

Exercise Technique

1. Exhale as you extend the arm straight back, lifting the weight until your arm is extended straight, feeling the tension in the back of the arm.

2. Lower the arm back to start position in a controlled manner.

REPEAT 8 TO 12 TIMES ON ONE SIDE, THEN REPEAT ON THE OTHER SIDE.

Triceps Dip Off Step

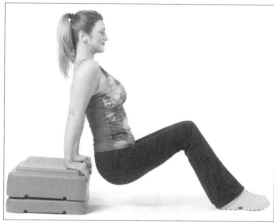

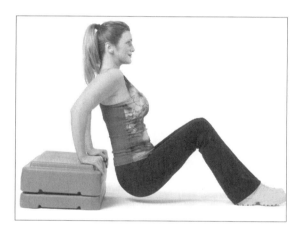

BODY PART WORKED
Back of Arms (Triceps)

SET UP
Sit on the long edge of a step with your hands gripping the edge of the step. Extend your legs out straight. Move your buttocks off the step and extend your arms straight.

TIPS FROM JONI
Keep your buttocks close to the step throughout the move.

Exercise Technique

1. Bend your elbows directly behind you, lowering your hips toward the floor, stopping before you feel any pressure in your shoulders.

2. Exhale as you push back up to start position until elbows are almost straight.

REPEAT 8 TO 12 TIMES.

CHAPTER 3
Shoulders and Arms

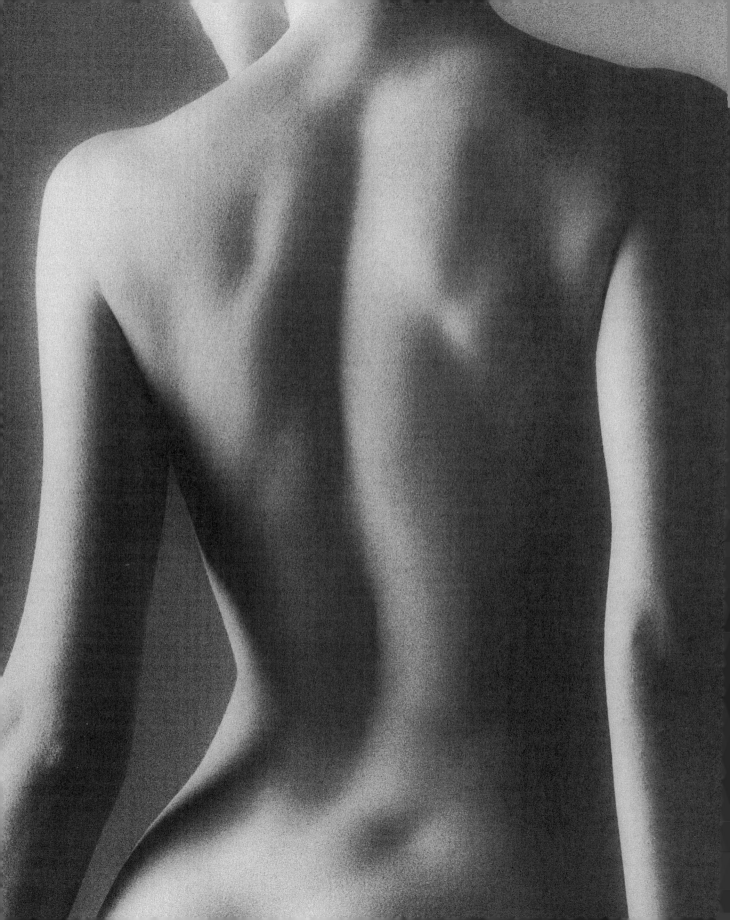

Chest and Back

The chest and upper back are often neglected, even by women who are experienced weight trainers. Many women focus on "mirror muscles" or parts of the body that they can see. Though this region seems unimportant, the core of your body cannot be ignored. The chest and upper back are opposing muscles that work together to enclose and protect crucial organs and assist in their function. Did you know that many back injuries and discomfort in the rest of the body can be prevented simply by strengthening the back muscles? A strong back also improves posture, and a trim and toned back provides a stunning rear view. From the front, although weight training does not increase your breast size, you can give them a lift by firming up the chest (pectoral) muscles that lie beneath the breasts. A natural and comfortable underwire!

ROUTINE A

BODY PART WORKED
Upper Back (Trapezius)

SET UP
Grip the bar just outside shoulder width with your palms facing toward you. Stand tall with feet just outside shoulder width. Both knees should be pointing straight ahead. Now bend forward at the hips with a slight bend in your knees. Your back should be straight, shoulders pulled back with your neck in line with your spine. The bar should be hanging straight down from your shoulders.

TIPS FROM JONI
Proper posture throughout this move is critical to back safety. Be aware of these posture positions during the entire exercise. Your back should be straight, abdominal muscles held in tightly, shoulders pulled back and your neck in line with your spine.

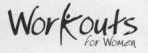

Bar Row To Chest

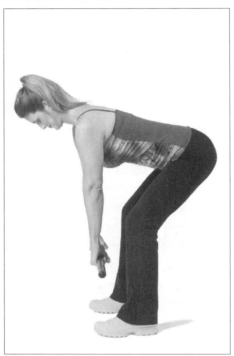
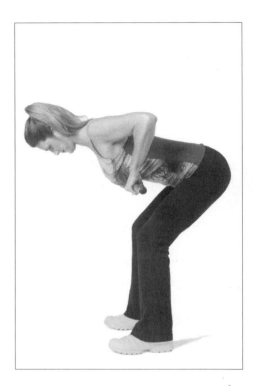

Exercise Technique
1. Exhale as you bend at the elbows, pulling the bar up toward your chest, squeezing your shoulder blades together at the top of the movement.

2. Lower the bar back down to start position.

REPEAT 8 TO 12 TIMES.

Seated Bent Over Rear Fly

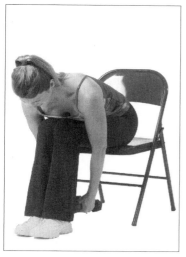 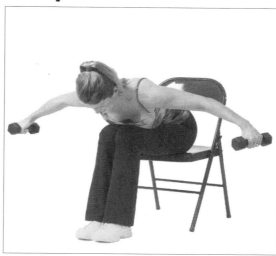

Exercise Technique

1. Exhale as you bend your arms at the elbows, pulling your hands up toward the ribcage, squeezing your shoulder blades together at the top of the move.

2. Reverse the move and lower your arms back to start position in a controlled manner.

REPEAT 8 TO 12 TIMES.

BODY PART WORKED
Upper Back (Trapezius)

SET UP
Hold a dumbbell in each hand and sit on the edge of a chair. Bend forward at the hips and hold your abdominal muscles in tight. Rest your chest on the thighs with your arms hanging at your sides, palms facing toward each other.

TIPS FROM JONI
Keep your back and neck in a straight line throughout the move.

CHAPTER 4
Chest and Back

31

ROUTINE A

BODY PART WORKED

Chest (Pectoral)

SET UP

Lie on top of the step with your neck and back supported. Start with your arms straight up, directly over your chest, with dumbbells in each hand and palms facing toward each other.

TIPS FROM JONI

Be sure not to let your back arch and lift off of the step as you lower the weight downward.

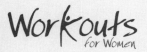

Chest Flies On Step

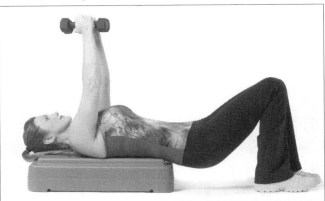

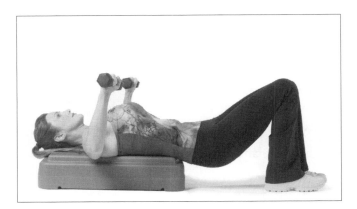

Exercise Technique

1. Bend arms at the elbows out in an arc as you lower the weight down, stopping when you feel a slight stretch through the chest.

2. Exhale and reverse the arc as you lift the weight back up to start position in a controlled manner.

REPEAT 8 TO 12 TIMES.

Bar Chest Press On Step

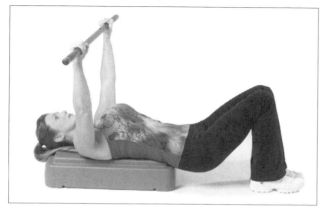

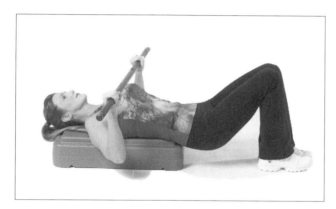

BODY PART WORKED

Chest (Pectoral)

SET UP

Grip a bar with a wide grip and lie on a step with your back and neck supported. Extend both arms straight up. The bar should be directly over your chest, with palms facing away from you.

TIPS FROM JONI

Be sure not to overextend the elbows at the top of the move.

Exercise Technique

1. Bend at the elbows as you lower the bar straight downward, stopping before the bar touches your chest.

2. Exhale as you extend your arms, pressing the weight straight back up to start position.

REPEAT 8 TO 12 TIMES.

CHAPTER 4
Chest and Back

BODY PART WORKED

Back (Latissimus Dorsi)

SET UP

Hold a bar with a shoulder width grip and lie on a step with your back and neck supported and both arms extended upward.

TIPS FROM JONI

Be sure not to let your back arch and come off of the step as you lower the weight behind you. Focus on keeping your pelvis tilted slightly upward, which will keep your back from arching by moving your spine down toward the step.

Bar Pullover On Step

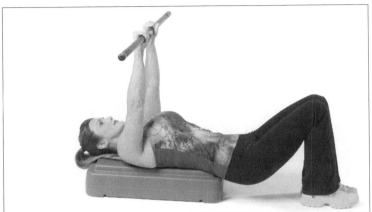

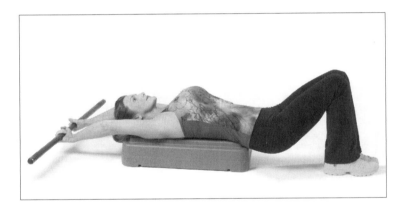

Exercise Technique

1. Keeping your arms almost straight and your back flat, lower the bar back and down overhead in an arc until you feel a slight stretch through your arms and chest.

2. Exhale and pull the weight back up to start position in a controlled manner.

REPEAT 8 TO 12 TIMES.

Workouts for Women

Bar Row To Ribs

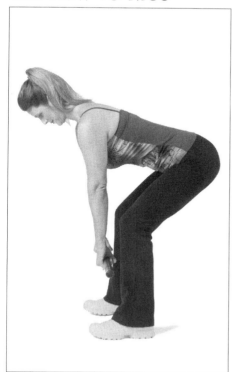 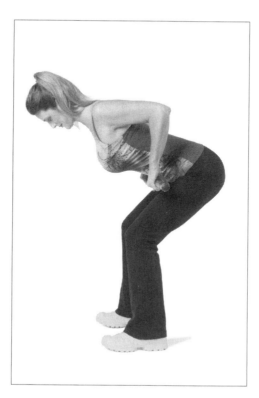

Exercise Technique

1. Exhale as you bend at the elbows, pulling the bar up toward your ribcage, squeezing your shoulder blades together at the top of the movement.

2. Lower the bar back down to start position.

REPEAT 8 TO 12 TIMES.

BODY PART WORKED
Mid-Back (Latissimus Dorsi, Rhomboid)

SET UP
Grip bar just outside shoulder width with your palms facing toward you. Stand tall with feet just outside shoulder width. Both knees should be pointing straight ahead. Bend forward at the hips with a slight bend in your knees. Your back should be straight, shoulders pulled back and neck in line with your spine. The bar should be hanging straight down from your shoulders.

TIPS FROM JONI
Proper posture throughout this move is critical to back safety. Your back should be straight, abdominal muscles held in tightly, shoulders pulled back and neck in line with your spine.

CHAPTER 4
Chest and Back

ROUTINE B

BODY PART WORKED
Mid-Back (Latissimus Dorsi)

SET UP
Begin this exercise in a semi-lunge position, standing with one leg forward and one back. Both knees should be pointing straight ahead and abdominal muscles should be held in tight. Lean forward, bending at the hip, and rest the forward hand on your forward thigh to support your body. Hold a dumbbell in the other hand and position the arm hanging down holding the weight near the forward knee.

TIPS FROM JONI
Be sure to keep your forward hand on the thigh to support your back throughout the move.

Workouts for Women

36

Bent Over Arc

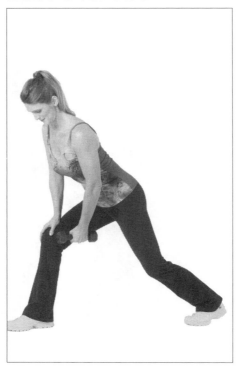 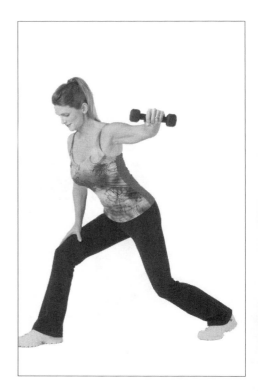

Exercise Technique

1. Exhale as you lift the weight out to the side in a wide arc, stopping at about shoulder height, squeezing the shoulder blades together at the top of the movement.

2. Reverse the arc, lowering the weight back down toward the forward knee and returning to start position.

REPEAT 8 TO 12 TIMES ON ONE SIDE, THEN THE OTHER.

Rotating Chest Press

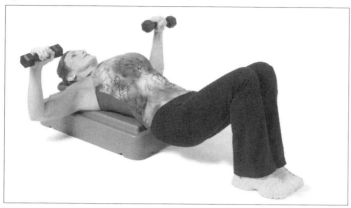

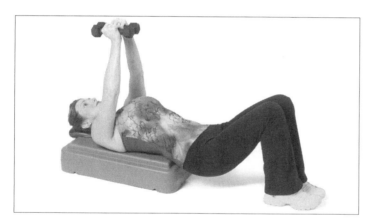

BODY PART WORKED

Chest (Pectoral)

SET UP

Lie on a step with your back flat and neck supported. Hold a dumbbell in each hand and bend arms at the elbows so that arms are in a goal post position with forearms parallel to the floor and palms facing away from you.

TIPS FROM JONI

Keep your wrists straight throughout the move.

Exercise Technique

1. Exhale as you press the weight up while rotating the palms of your hands in toward each other, bringing hands together at the top of the move.

2. Reverse the move and lower the weight, rotating your hands back out, stopping when your forearms are parallel to the floor.

REPEAT 8 TO 12 TIMES.

CHAPTER 4
Chest and Back

ROUTINE B

BODY PART WORKED

Back (Latissimus Dorsi)

SET UP

Lie on the step with your back and neck supported and both arms extended upward with a dumbbell in each hand.

TIPS FROM JONI

Be sure not to let your back arch and come off of the step as you lower the weight behind you.

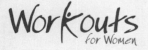

Straight Arm Pullover On Step

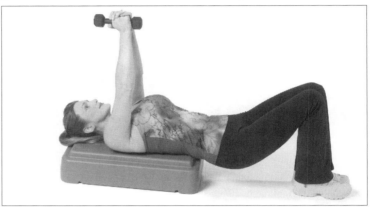

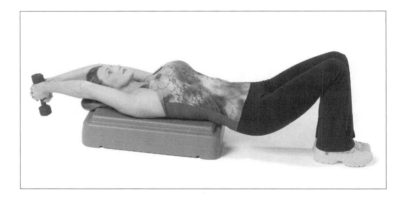

Exercise Technique

1. Keeping your arms almost straight and your back flat, lower the weight back and down over your head in an arc until you feel a slight stretch through your arms and chest.

2. Exhale and pull the weight back up to start position in a controlled manner.

REPEAT 8 TO 12 TIMES.

Wide Grip Push-Ups

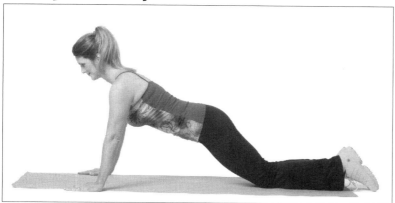

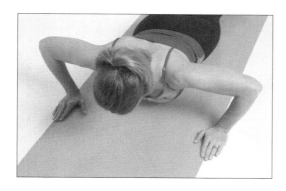

Exercise Technique

1. Bend your elbows and lower your chest, stopping one fist distance from the floor.

2. Exhale as you push your body back up to start position.

REPEAT 8 TO 12 TIMES.

BODY PART WORKED
Chest (Pectoral)

SET UP
Get on your hands and knees with hands placed outside shoulder width, fingers facing forward and knees extended back as far as comfortable. Hold your abdominal muscles in tight.

TIPS FROM JONI
Keep elbows soft (slightly bent) as you extend back up to start position. Keep abdominal muscles tight and your neck in line with your spine at all times.
To decrease the difficulty of the move, bring your hands and knees in closer together.

CHAPTER 4
Chest and Back

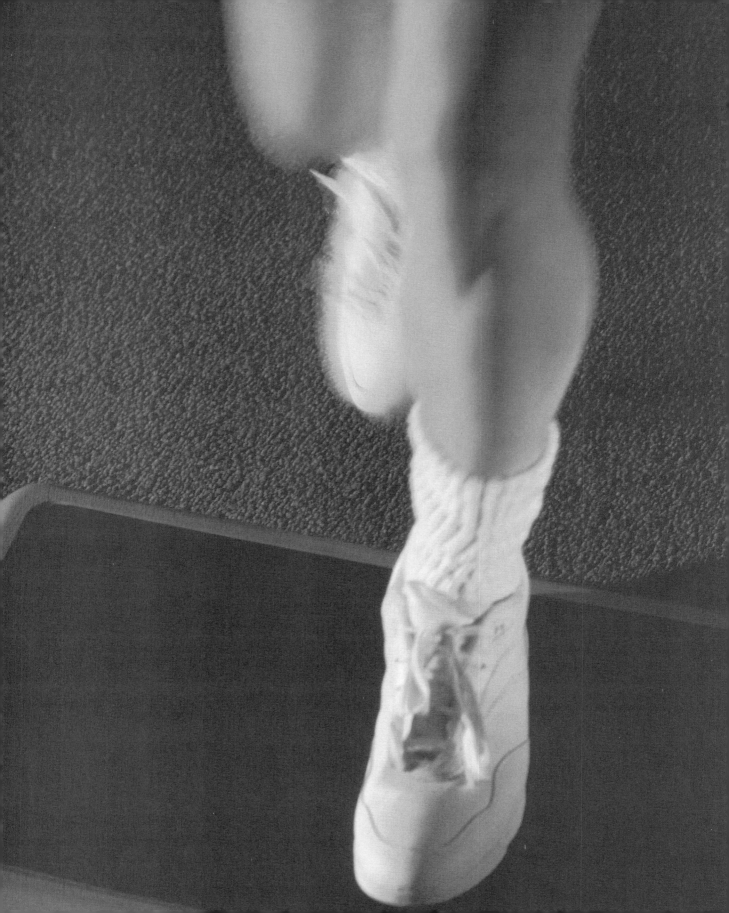

Lower Body

The lower body, consisting of legs, buttocks, hips and thighs, is a hot Zone altogether. This is a Zone that literally keeps you going year after year. We bend, reach, lift, twist, lean, run, walk, and sit in the name of household chores, child care, work, recreational activities and LIFE. Not one of the muscles in this group is left unused throughout the day. This Zone gives us power. Unfortunately, it is not your imagination that for many women every extra calorie goes straight to the lower body. Creating more lean muscle in the lower body is key to long-term weight control. Since some of the largest muscle groups are in our lower body, focusing on this area will create a body that efficiently burns fat 24/7. This Zone Workout will tighten the buttocks (gluteus maximus) and trim the hips and thighs. In addition, it will sculpt the front (quadriceps) and back (hamstrings) of your legs, creating sleek, well-toned legs.

ROUTINE A

BODY PART WORKED

Inner Thigh (Adductor)

SET UP

Grip a weighted bar with palms facing out. Carefully lift the bar up so you are holding it close to your body right above your chest. Stand with your abdominal muscles held in tight, shoulders back and chest high with legs double shoulder width apart. Point your toes and knees out-ward.

TIPS FROM JONI

To keep the focus of the move on the inner thigh, keep your buttocks tucked under and keep your knees pressing back.

Weighted Pliés

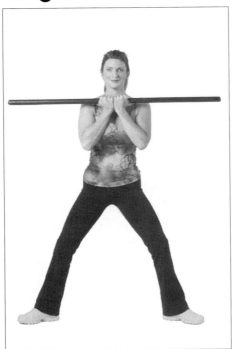 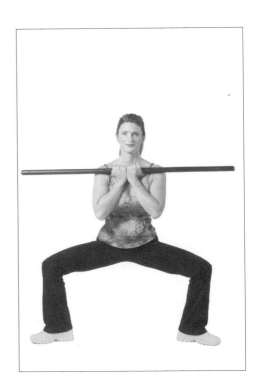

Exercise Technique

1. Bend at the knees, lowering your hips toward the floor, stopping when you feel a stretch in the inner thigh.

2. Exhale and press through your heels, straightening your legs and returning back to starting position.

REPEAT 8 TO 12 TIMES.

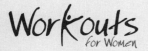

Weighted Walking Lunge

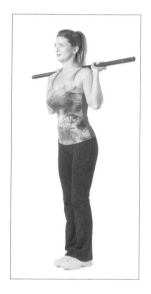 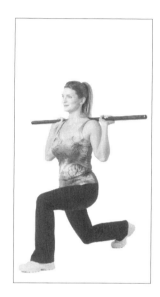 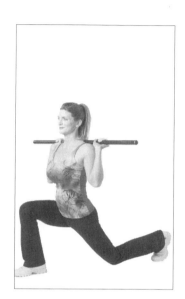

Exercise Technique

1. Take a long step forward with one leg, landing first with the heel.

2. As that forward foot impacts the floor, immediately bend at the knees, lowering your hips toward the floor.

3. Push off with the ball of the rear foot as you take a step forward so that now you are standing tall with feet together again.

REPEAT A TOTAL OF 20 TIMES, ALTERNATING RIGHT AND LEFT LEGS.

BODY PART WORKED

Front of Thighs, Buttocks (Quadriceps, Gluteus Maximus)

SET UP

Grip a bar with palms facing in and carefully raise it over your head, bringing it down to rest on top of your shoulders behind your neck. Stand up straight with legs together and shoulders back, chest high and abdominal muscles held in tight.

TIPS FROM JONI

Be careful not to lock your knees as you return to start. As you lower, be sure that your front knee stays directly over your ankle and does not move past your toes. If you have difficulty with balance, do not use the weighted bar. Keep your elbows rotated forward throughout the move to assist in keeping proper posture.

CHAPTER 5
Lower Body

ROUTINE A

BODY PART WORKED
Buttocks (Gluteus Maximus)

SET UP
Grip a bar with palms facing in and carefully raise it over your head, bringing it down to rest on top of your shoulders behind your neck. Stand with feet just outside shoulder width, abdominal muscles held in tight, shoulders back, chest high and toes pointing straight ahead.

TIPS FROM JONI
Be careful not to lock your knees as you return to start. As you lower, be sure that your front knees stay directly over your ankles and do not move past your toes. Keep your elbows rotated forward throughout the move to assist in keeping proper posture.

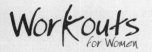

Weighted Squats

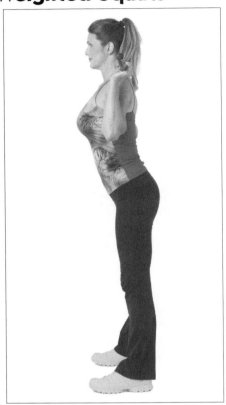 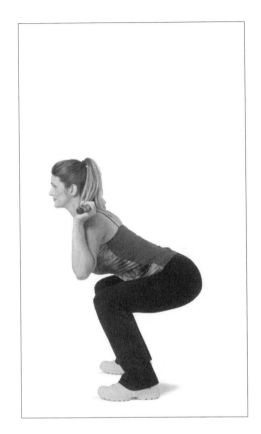

Exercise Technique

1. Begin this exercise by bending at the knees and reach back with your buttocks as if you were sitting onto a chair behind you.

2. Stop when your hips are knee level. Do not drop any lower.

3. Exhale as you press yourself back up to standing position with the majority of your weight pressing up through your heels.

4. Contract the buttocks at the top of the move as you stand back up.

REPEAT 8 TO 12 TIMES.

Mule Kick

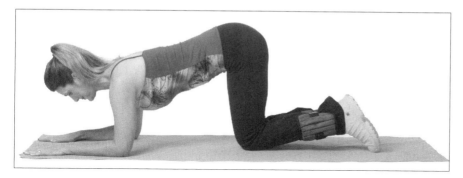

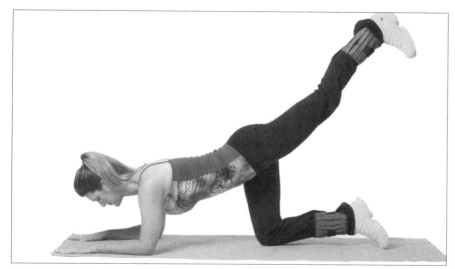

BODY PART WORKED
Buttocks (Gluteus Maximus)

SET UP
With ankle weights around each leg, get down on your knees and forearms with abdominal muscles held in tight.

TIPS FROM JONI
Keep your neck in a relaxed position. Keep both hips square to the floor during the entire movement.

Exercise Technique

1. With your foot flexed, exhale as you kick up and out with one leg, squeezing the buttocks at the top of the motion when your leg is extended.

2. Bend your leg at the knee, pulling it back into start position without resting your knee on the floor.

REPEAT 8 TO 12 TIMES ON ONE SIDE, THEN REPEAT ON THE OPPOSITE.

CHAPTER 5
Lower Body

ROUTINE A

BODY PART WORKED

Outer Thigh (Abductor)

SET UP

With ankle weights on each leg, lie on the floor on your side with the top arm in front of your body supporting your weight. Hips and legs should be directly on top of each other with both legs extended straight.

TIPS FROM JONI

Be sure that hips stay stacked directly on top of each other throughout the move

Lying Straight Leg Outer Thigh

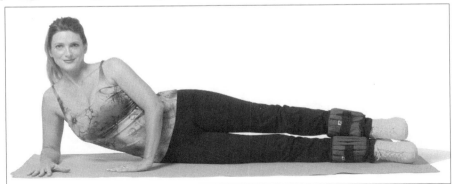

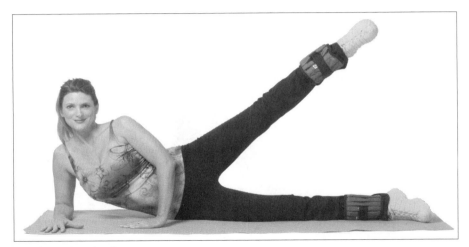

Exercise Technique

1. Exhale and lead with the heel as you lift the top leg as high as you comfortably can.

2. Lower the leg back down in a controlled manner without resting it on the other leg. Repeat.

REPEAT 8 TO 12 TIMES ON ONE SIDE, THEN ON THE OPPOSITE.

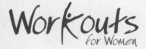

Weighted Squats Side-to-Side

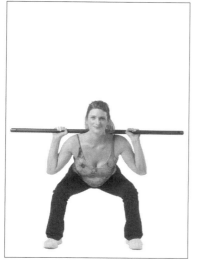 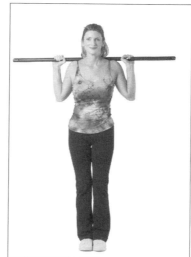

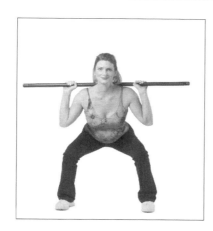

BODY PART WORKED
Hips and Buttocks, Inner and Outer Thigh (Gluteus Maximus, Adductor, Abductor)

SET UP
Grip a bar with palms facing forward and carefully raise it over your head, bringing it down to rest on top of your shoulders behind your neck. Stand tall with feet together and abdominal muscles held in tight, shoulders back, chest high and toes pointing straight ahead.

TIPS FROM JONI
Be careful not to lock your knees as you return to start position. As you lower, be sure that your knees stay directly over your ankles and do not move past your toes. Keep your elbows rotated forward throughout the move to assist in keeping proper posture.

Exercise Technique
1. Begin this exercise by bending at the knees as you step out directly to the side with one leg, reaching back with your buttocks as if you were sitting back onto a chair behind you.

2. Stop when your hips are knee level. Do not drop any lower.

3. Exhale as you press yourself back up to standing position with the majority of your weight pressing up through your heels.

4. Contract the buttocks at the top of the move as you stand back up.

REPEAT A TOTAL OF 20 TIMES, ALTERNATING SIDE TO SIDE.

CHAPTER 5
Lower Body

BODY PART WORKED

Thighs (Adductor, Abductor, Quadricep)

SET UP

Stand up straight with shoulders back, chest high and abdominal muscles held in tight. Now, establish a correct lunge position.

TIPS FROM JONI

Be careful not to lock your knees as you return to start position.

As you lower, be sure that your front knee stays directly over your ankle and does not move past your toes. Position a chair next to you to hold onto for balance.

Keep your elbows rotated forward throughout the move to assist in keeping proper posture.

For an added challenge, position a weighted bar on your shoulders.

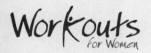

Stationary Lunge

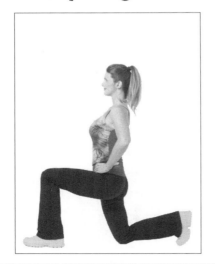
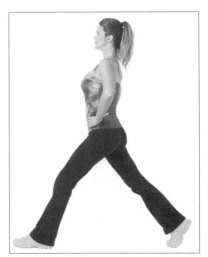

To Find the Correct Lunge Position: Kneel down. Step one leg forward with the heel directly above the ankle. Now stand up. Your legs should be shoulder width apart and the heel of the rear foot should be up. Pull your shoulders back, chest out and hold your abdominal muscles in tight.

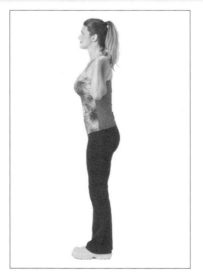
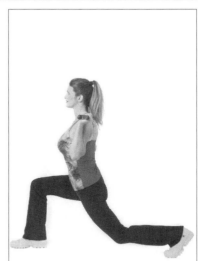

Exercise Technique

1. Bend both knees and lower your hips toward the floor, stopping before your back knee touches the ground.

2. Exhale as you straighten your knees and press yourself up with the heel of your forward foot and the toes of your back foot, lifting your body straight up to start position.

REPEAT 8 TO 12 TIMES ON EACH SIDE.

Weighted Alternating Reverse Lunge

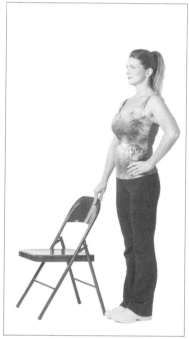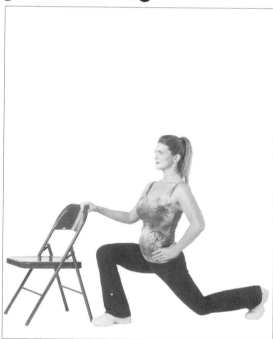

BODY PART WORKED
Front of Thighs and Back of Thighs (Quadriceps and Hamstrings)

SET UP
Grip a bar with palms facing in and carefully raise it over your head, bringing it down to rest on top of your shoulders behind your neck. Stand up straight and tall with legs together, shoulders back, chest high and abdomen held in tight.

TIPS FROM JONI
As you lower down, the front knee should always be directly over your ankle and should not extend past your toes or you will be placing too much pressure on the knee.

If you have difficulty with balance, do not use the weighted bar. Also, position a chair next to you to hold onto for balance.

Keep your elbows rotated forward throughout the move which will assist in keeping proper posture.

Exercise Technique

1. Take a slow, controlled step back with one leg, landing on the ball of the foot.

2. Bend both knees, lowering your hips toward the floor, stopping before the back knee touches the floor.

3. Exhale as you push off the trailing foot and the front heel as you straighten your legs, returning to start position.

Note: Pictured is the exercise for those with balance difficulties. To see how a bar should be held, see page 67.

REPEAT 20 TIMES.

CHAPTER 5
Lower Body

ROUTINE B

BODY PART WORKED

Inner Thigh (Adductor)

SET UP

Lie on your side with your bottom leg extended and the top leg bent with foot flat on the floor behind the bottom leg. Shift your body weight onto the lower hip and prop your body up with the corresponding forearm.

TIPS FROM JONI

It's important to keep the heel of the extended leg rotated upward to keep the focus on the inner thigh.

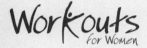

Inner Thigh Lift

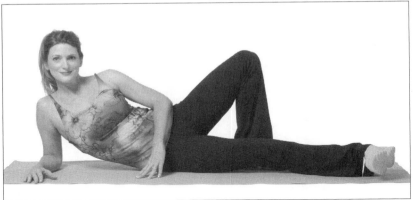

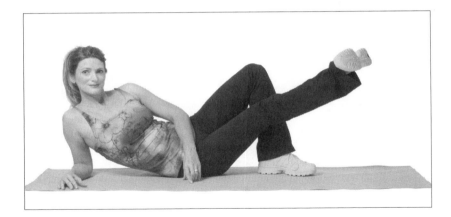

Exercise Technique

1. With the foot flexed and heel rotated upward, exhale and lift the extended leg upward as high as you can comfortably go.

2. Lower the leg back down in a controlled manner without touching the floor.

REPEAT 8 TO 12 TIMES ON ONE SIDE, THEN REPEAT ON THE OPPOSITE.

Kneeling Straight Leg Glute

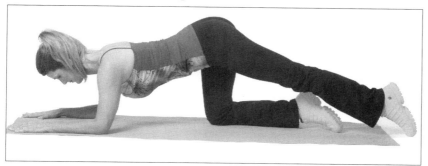

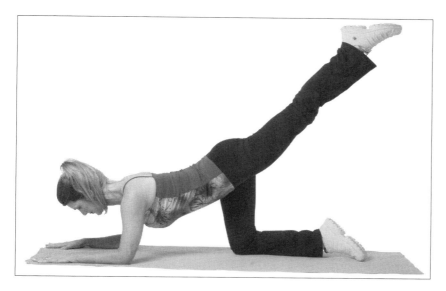

BODY PART WORKED
Buttocks (Gluteus Maximus)

SET UP
Get on your elbows and knees. Extend one leg back with toes pointed. Hold your abdominal muscles in tight.

TIPS FROM JONI
Keep hips square to the floor throughout the move.

Exercise Technique

1. Exhale as you lift the extended leg up as high as possible, squeezing the buttocks at the top of the move.

2. Bring the extended leg back down, momentarily tapping your toes lightly on the floor.

REPEAT 8 TO 12 TIMES ON ONE SIDE, THEN REPEAT ON THE OPPOSITE.

CHAPTER 5
Lower Body

51

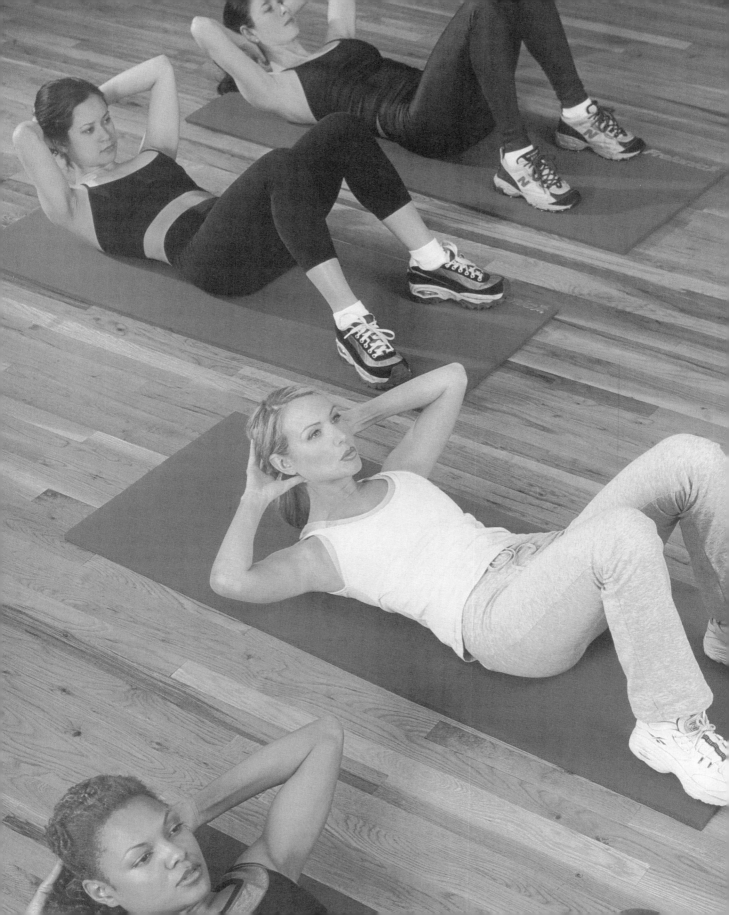

Abdominals and Lower Back

The abdominal muscles and the muscles of the lower back are opposing muscle groups. In addition to core strength, women simply want to have a sexy midsection. The abdominals are a stubborn part of your body, prone to fat storage. Other parts of your body, such as your legs, show results and muscle tone much more quickly. It is not easy to achieve a perfectly flat abdomen, and in some cases it is impossible. However, everyone can greatly improve the abdominal area. And strengthening the lower back muscles can help you shape up all the way around. This Zone Workout is designed to strengthen and tone the muscles of the abdomen (rectus abdominis), the lateral torso muscles (obliques) and the muscles of your lower back (erector spinae). Look forward to wearing clothes that will show off your incredible midsection.

Technical Notes For Exercising Your Abdominal Muscles

Optimal results in training the abdominal muscles are achieved if you train them until fatigue, or until you can do no more. You are not limited to a prescribed number of abdominal exercises, but rather continue until you feel yourself compromising form or you can do no more. For instance, if your abdominal muscles are not fatigued with 20 or 30 repetitions of crunches, then continue. Just keep in mind, 10 or 20 well-executed crunches are more beneficial than 50 sloppy ones. Here are more tips for effective abdominal exercises:

1. When you perform your abdominal exercises, focus on the exact area that is being worked. It is easy to allow other muscles to do some of the work and therefore not get the full and proper benefit of an exercise. If you allow your neck or hip flexors to help you out, your abdominal muscles will not get fatigued or toned.

2. Practicing proper breathing technique is especially important when working your abdominals. This is done by exhaling on the exertion, which is when you

lift up. This decreases internal air pressure, allowing you to fully involve the abdominal muscles.

3. Train your abdominal muscles by keeping them contracted when performing all your other exercises and also when sitting, standing or driving. Consciously holding them in can reduce back strain and help to flatten your entire midsection.

4. You cannot overtrain your abdominal muscles. It is acceptable to do a few sets of abdominal exercises every day.

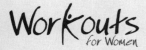

Dead Lift

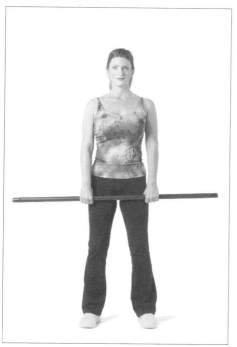 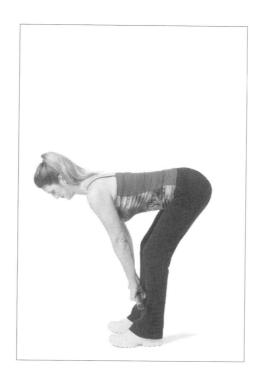

Exercise Technique

1. Bend forward at the hips with a slight bend in your knees, reaching back with your tailbone and allowing your hands to move downward toward your feet. Your back should be straight, abdominal muscles held in tight, shoulders pulled back and neck in line with your spine.

2. Stop at the point at which you feel slight tension in the back of your legs, then exhale as you stand back up, returning to start.

REPEAT 8 TO 12 TIMES.

BODY PART WORKED

Back of Legs/Lower Back (Hamstring, Erector Spinae)

SET UP

Grip weighted bar just outside shoulder width with your palms facing toward you. Stand tall and position your feet loosely together, with hands and arms hanging straight down at your sides.

TIPS FROM JONI

Keep the weighted bar very close to your body throughout the entire move to prevent strain on the lower back.

Follow proper posture throughout the move to protect your back: Your back should be straight, abdominal muscles held in tight, shoulders pulled back and neck in line with your spine.

CHAPTER 6
Abdominals and Lower Back

ROUTINE A

BODY PART WORKED
Upper and Lower Abdomen (Rectus Abdominis)

SET UP
Lie flat on your back with your knees bent, heels close to your body and pelvis tilted slightly upward to help flatten your back. Place your fingertips lightly on the back of your head.

TIPS FROM JONI
Focus on moving your rib-cage toward your hip bone as you lift up. Keep your elbows back and out of sight. Keep your chin one fist distance off your chest.

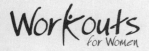

Knee Up Crunches

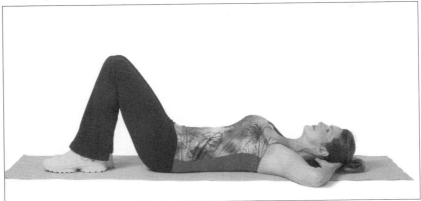

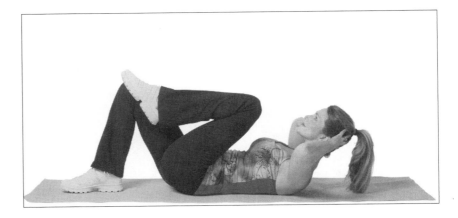

Exercise Technique

1. Exhale as you lift your shoulder blades up and forward while simultaneously bringing one knee up and in toward your chest.

2. Lower your leg back down to start position and repeat on the other side without resting your head on the floor.

REPEAT UNTIL FATIGUED.

Oblique Pulses

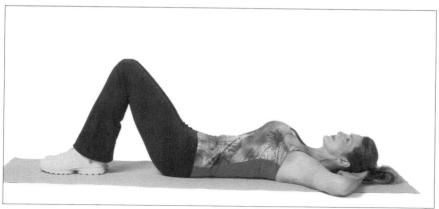

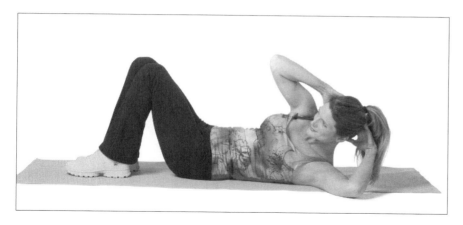

Exercise Technique

1. Exhale as you lift and rotate one shoulder toward the opposite knee.

2. Lower your shoulder back down to start position, then immediately perform the move on the opposite side.

3. Perform this move in a fast-paced pulsing motion, alternating from side to side.

REPEAT UNTIL FATIGUED.

BODY PART WORKED
Sides of Waist (Obliques)

SET UP
Lie on your back with knees bent and heels close to your body. Tilt the pelvis up slightly to flatten out your back. Place fingertips lightly on the back of your head.

TIPS FROM JONI
Be sure not to compromise your form on this move due to the faster pace.

CHAPTER 6
Abdominals and Lower Back

ROUTINE A

BODY PART WORKED

Lower Abdomen (Rectus Abdominis)

SET UP

Lie on your back with your hands under the buttocks to lift the pelvis up slightly and flatten the back. Lift both legs up with knees bent to a 90 degree angle.

TIPS FROM JONI

Concentrate on using your abdominal muscles and not momentum to perform this move.

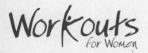

Bicycles

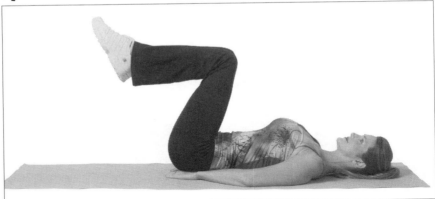

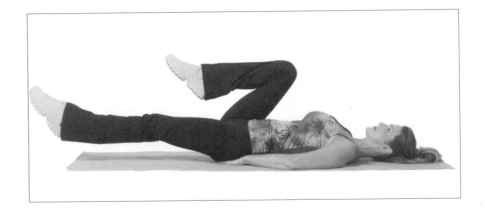

Exercise Technique

1. Exhale as you extend one leg out straight and parallel to the floor, as the opposite knee simultaneously bends and comes in toward your chest.

ALTERNATE FROM SIDE TO SIDE UNTIL FATIGUED.

Plank

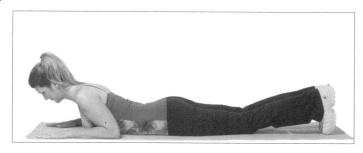

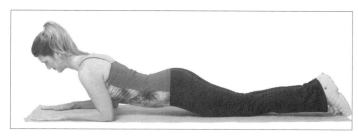

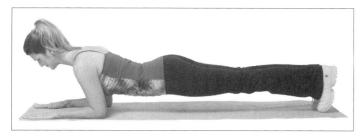

Exercise Technique

1. Exhale as you lift your midsection up off the floor and rise up onto your knees first, then up to your toes and forearms, keeping your back and buttocks at a flat angle from knees to shoulders.

2. Hold this position for 5 seconds.

3. Slowly and carefully come back down onto your knees, and move right back into Set Up position, resting for 5 seconds before lifting up again.

REPEAT UNTIL FATIGUED.

ROUTINE A

BODY PART WORKED
Core Muscles, Including Trunk and Pelvis (Rectus Abdominis and Transverse Abdominis)

SET UP
Lie face down on the floor with your elbows bent and hands next to your chest, palms facing down.

TIPS FROM JONI
During the 5 second holding phase, a common tendency is to hold your breath. Be sure to breathe normally throughout the move.

CHAPTER 6
Abdominals and Lower Back

ROUTINE B

BODY PART WORKED

Upper and Lower Abdomen (Rectus Abdominis)

SET UP

Lie flat on your back with a weighted bar resting on top of your chest. Your knees should be bent, heels close to your body and pelvis tilted slightly upward to help flatten your back.

TIPS FROM JONI

Focus on moving your ribcage toward your hip bone as you lift up.
Keep your chin one fist distance off your chest.

Weighted Crunch

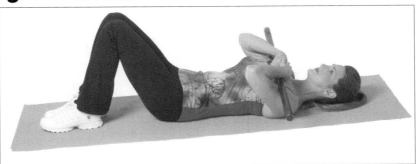

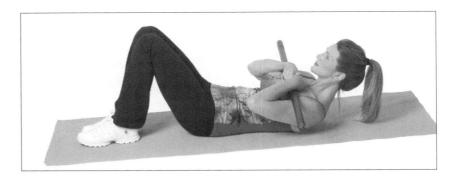

Exercise Technique

1. Exhale as you lift your upper back and shoulders up and forward.

2. Reverse the move, lowering your upper back and shoulders toward the floor but not resting your head on the floor.

REPEAT UNTIL FATIGUED.

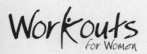

Reverse Curl

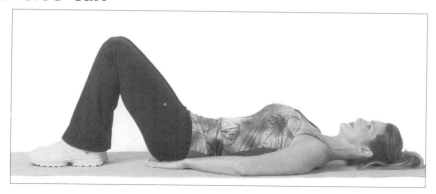

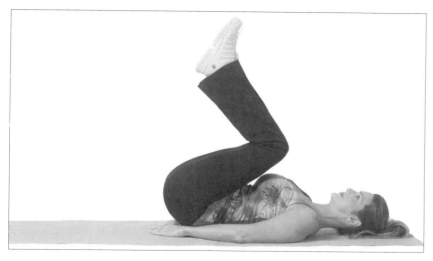

BODY PART WORKED
Lower Abdomen (Rectus Abdominis)

SET UP
Lie on your back with your hands under the buttocks to lift the pelvis up slightly and flatten the back. Place your feet flat on the floor with your knees bent.

TIPS FROM JONI
Be sure not to rock your body to lift your legs up. Use your abdominal muscles to lift your pelvis and buttocks, which will keep the focus on the lower abdominal muscles.

Exercise Technique

1. Keeping knees bent and together, exhale as you lift the pelvis and buttocks up off the floor, bringing your knees in toward the chest.

2. Keeping knees bent and together, reverse the move by rolling the pelvis and buttocks back toward the floor. As your feet come back toward the floor, momentarily tap your toes onto the floor and then repeat the move.

REPEAT UNTIL FATIGUED.

CHAPTER 6
Abdominals and Lower Back

ROUTINE B

BODY PART WORKED
Sides of Waist (Oblique)

SET UP
Lie on your back with knees bent and heels close to your body. Tilt the pelvis up slightly to flatten out your back. Place fingertips lightly on the back of your head.

TIPS FROM JONI
The lifting and rotating motion really focuses on the waist. Complete each move with precision and focus for maximum results.

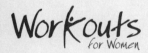

Knee In Oblique

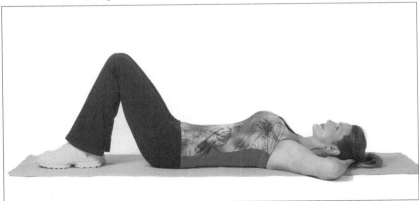

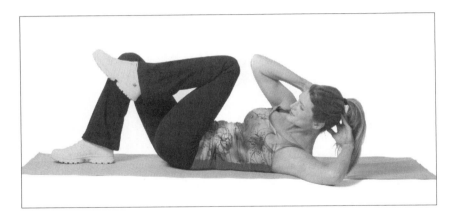

Exercise Technique

1. Exhale as you lift and rotate one shoulder toward the opposite knee as you simultaneously lift that opposite knee toward the shoulder.

2. Lower shoulder and knee back down to start position, then immediately perform the move on the opposite side.

ALTERNATE FROM SIDE TO SIDE UNTIL FATIGUED.

Reach Crunch

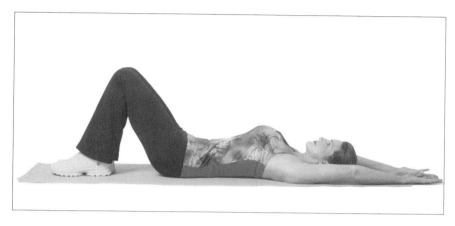

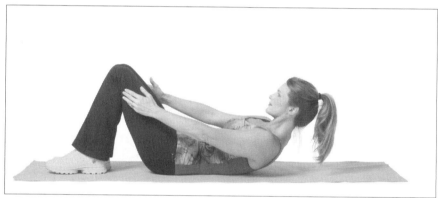

Exercise Technique

1. Exhale as you lift your shoulders and upper back off the floor, bringing your arms over your body in an arc, reaching toward your feet.

2. Reverse the move, lowering your upper back and shoulders toward the floor with your arms extended straight overhead, but not resting your head on the floor.

REPEAT UNTIL FATIGUED.

ROUTINE B

BODY PART WORKED
Upper Abdomen (Rectus Abdominis)

SET UP
Lie flat on your back with your knees bent, heels close to your body and pelvis tilted slightly upward to help flatten the back. Extend your arms overhead.

TIPS FROM JONI
Keep your chin one fist distance off your chest throughout the move.

CHAPTER 6
Abdominals and Lower Back

ROUTINE B

BODY PART WORKED

Lower Back (Erector Spinae)

SET UP

Lie face down with your legs extended and arms extended overhead.

TIPS FROM JONI

This is a great move to strengthen the lower back. Perform this move smoothly, flowing into the position.

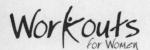

Superwoman

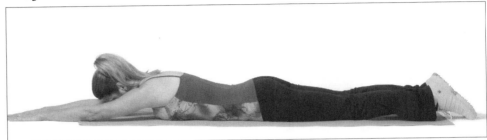

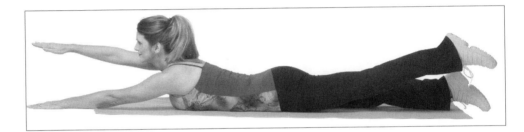

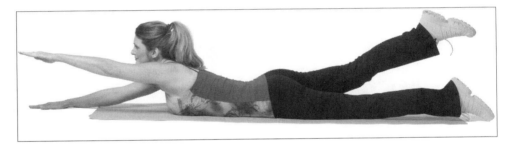

Exercise Technique

1. Exhale as you lift the opposite arm and opposite leg simultaneously, holding for a moment.

2. Slowly lower back to start position and smoothly follow with the same motion using the opposite arm and leg.

REPEAT A TOTAL OF 8 TO 12 TIMES, ALTERNATING RIGHT AND LEFT.

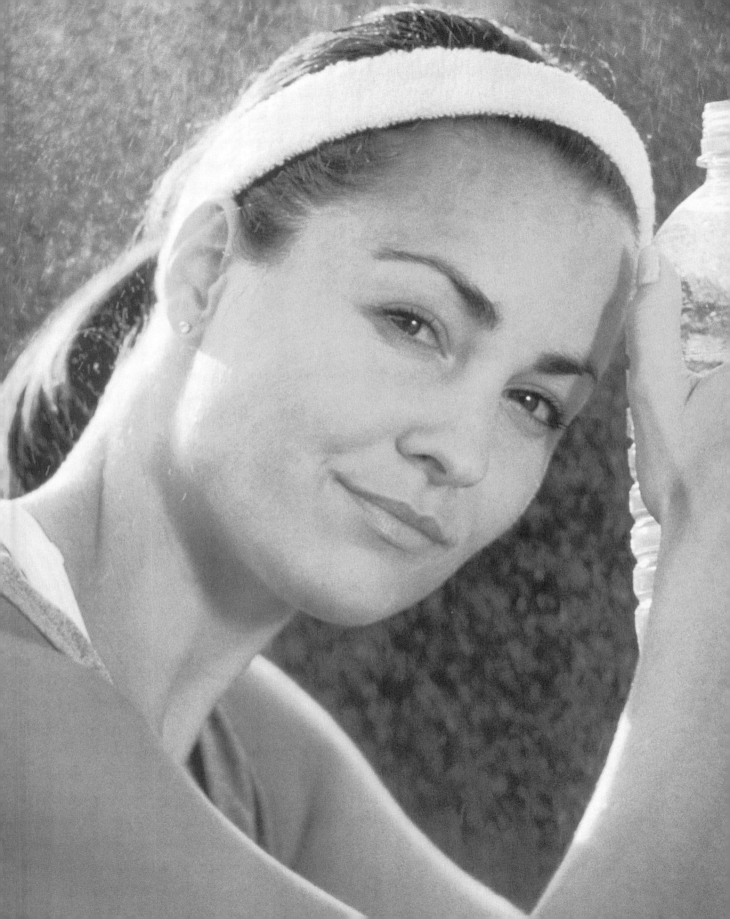

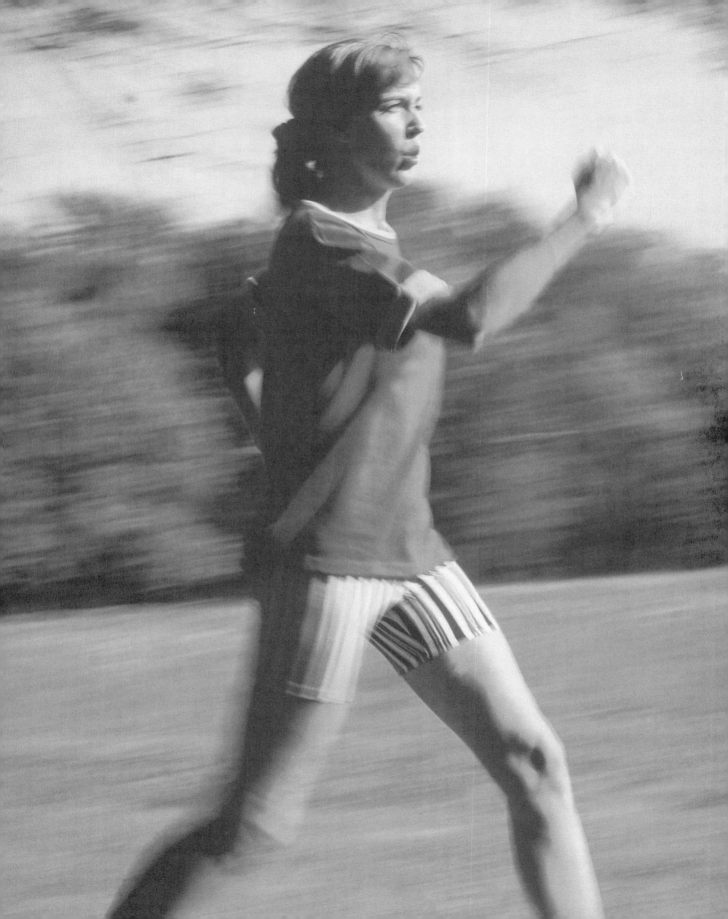

CHAPTER 7

Total Body

Tight and toned muscles can offer you a slimmer look without losing an ounce. However, you are increasing overall lean muscle mass, which will fire up your metabolism and burn extra calories, resulting in weight loss. This is the most effective way to gain long-term weight control. This total body workout will hit all the Zones in one efficient routine and help you to defy the laws of gravity by giving your body a lift! Weight training is a proven way to burn calories, build and preserve bone density, and help prevent heart disease as you create new curves.

ROUTINE A

BODY PART WORKED

Hips and Buttocks, Inner and Outer Thigh (Gluteus Maximus, Adductor, Abductor)

SET UP

Grip a bar with palms facing forward and carefully raise it over your head, bringing it down to rest on top of your shoulders behind your neck. Stand with feet just outside shoulder width, shoulders back, chest high and toes pointing straight ahead.

TIPS FROM JONI

Be careful not to lock your knees as you return to start position. As you lower down, be sure that your knees stay directly over your ankles and do not move past your toes. Keep your elbows rotated forward throughout the move. As you lift your leg out to the side, go only as high as you can without compromising your posture.

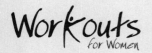

Weighted Squats and Side Lift

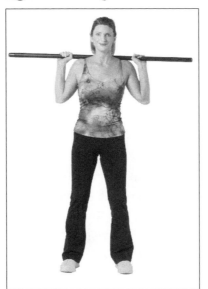
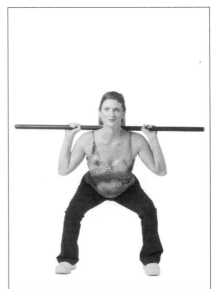
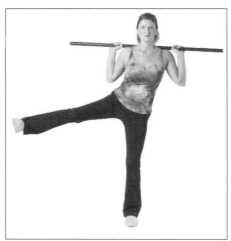

Exercise Technique

1. Begin this exercise by bending at the knees and reach back with your buttocks as if you were sitting back onto a chair behind you.

2. Stop when your hips are knee level. Do not drop any lower.

3. Exhale as you press yourself back up to standing position with the majority of your weight pressing up through your heels and simultaneously bring one leg up and out directly to the side.

4. Control the leg as you lower it, bringing it back in, and smoothly sit back down in a squat.

REPEAT 20 TIMES, ALTERNATING SIDES.

Weighted Forward Lunge

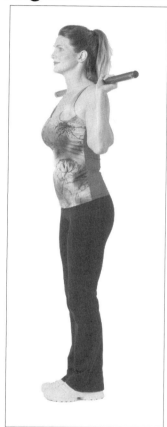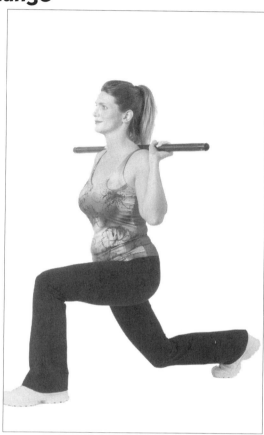

Exercise Technique

1. Take a long step forward with one leg, landing first with the heel.

2. As that forward foot impacts the floor, immediately bend at the knees, lowering your hips toward the floor.

3. Push off the front heel and return to start.

REPEAT A TOTAL OF 20 TIMES, ALTERNATING RIGHT AND LEFT.

BODY PART WORKED

Front of Thighs, Buttocks (Quadriceps, Gluteus Maximus)

SET UP

Grip a bar with palms facing forward and carefully raise it over your head, bringing it down to rest on top of your shoulders behind your neck. Stand up straight with legs together and shoulders back, chest high and abdominal muscles held in tight.

TIPS FROM JONI

Be careful not to lock your knees as you return to start position. As you lower down, be sure that your front knee stays directly over your ankle and does not move past your toes. If you have difficulty with balance, do not use the weighted bar. Also, position a chair next to you to hold onto for balance. Keep your elbows rotated forward throughout the move to assist in keeping proper posture.

CHAPTER 7
Total Body

ROUTINE A

BODY PART WORKED

Front of Arms (Bicep)

SET UP

Stand tall with shoulders back, chest high and abdominal muscles held in tight. Hold a dumbbell in each hand and stand with feet about shoulder width apart. Place your arms down at your sides with the palms facing in.

TIPS FROM JONI

Keep elbows stationary at your sides throughout the move, being sure they do not move forward or backward.

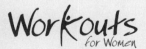

Hammer Curls

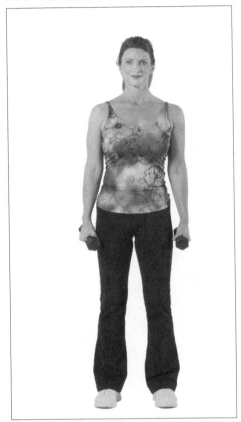 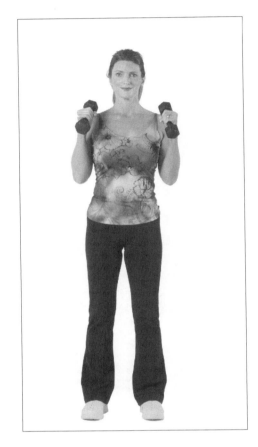

Exercise Technique

1. Exhale as you bend your arms at the elbows, lifting your hands up toward your shoulders.

2. Extend arms back down to your sides in a controlled manner.

REPEAT 8 TO 12 TIMES.

Bent Over Tricep Kickback

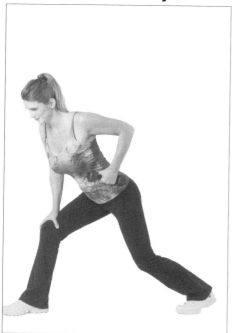 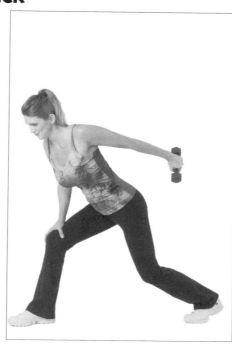

Exercise Technique

1. Exhale as you extend the arm straight back, lifting the weight until your arm is extended straight, feeling the tension in the back of the arm.

2. Lower the arm back to start in a controlled manner.

REPEAT 8 TO 12 TIMES ON ONE SIDE, THEN REPEAT ON THE OPPOSITE.

BODY PART WORKED

Back of Upper Arm (Tricep)

SET UP

Begin this exercise in a semi-lunge position, standing with one leg forward and one back. Both knees should be pointing straight ahead and abdominal muscles should be held in tight. Lean forward, bending at the hip, and rest the forward hand on your forward thigh to support your body. Hold a dumbbell in the other hand and raise the arm up and bend at the elbow, so that the upper arm is in line with your torso and close to your body.

TIPS FROM JONI

Keep your elbow stationary and close to your body throughout the move. Be sure not to swing the working arm. Concentrate on using the muscles in the back of your arm to lift the weight.

CHAPTER 7
Total Body

ROUTINE A

BODY PART WORKED

Front of Shoulders (Medial Deltoid)

SET UP

Holding dumbbells in both hands, stand tall with abdominal muscles held in tight, shoulders back and chest high. Start with both arms in front of your body, bent at the elbows so that hands are shoulder height with palms facing forward. Upper arms should be parallel to the floor.

TIPS FROM JONI

Keep elbows in front of your body throughout the move to keep the focus on the front of the shoulders.

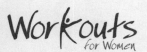

Military Press

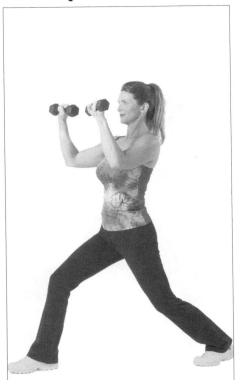 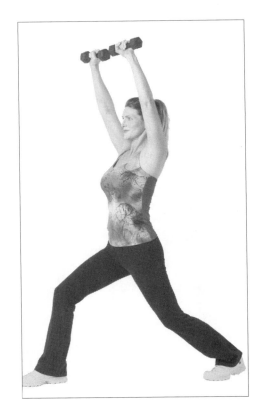

Exercise Technique

1. Exhale as you extend arms straight overhead.

2. Bend at the elbows as you lower back to start position.

REPEAT 8 TO 12 TIMES.

Seated Bent Over Rear Fly

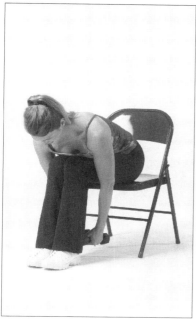 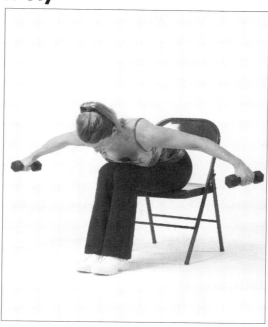

BODY PART WORKED

Upper Back (Trapezius)

SET UP

Hold a dumbbell in each hand and sit on the edge of a chair. Bend forward at the hips. Rest your chest on your thighs with your arms hanging at your side, palms facing toward each other.

TIPS FROM JONI

Be sure not to use momentum during this move. Focus on using your back muscles during the lifting phase.

Exercise Technique

1. Exhale as you bend arms at the elbows, pulling your hands up toward the ribcage. Squeeze your shoulder blades together at the top of the move.

2. Reverse the move and lower your arms back to start position in a controlled manner.

REPEAT 8 TO 12 TIMES.

CHAPTER 7
Total Body

ROUTINE A

BODY PART WORKED

Outer Thigh (Abductor)

SET UP

With ankle weights around each leg, stand next to a chair with a slight bend in the knees, holding on to the chair for balance. Keep your abdominal muscles held in tight, shoulders back and chest high.

TIPS FROM JONI

Keeping the toes rotated forward forces you to lift with the heel and keeps the focus of this exercise on the outer thigh.

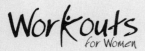

Standing Outer Thigh

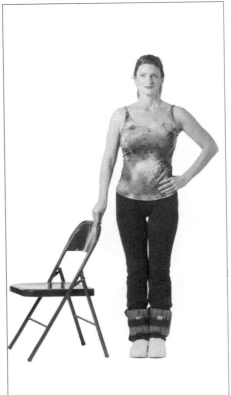
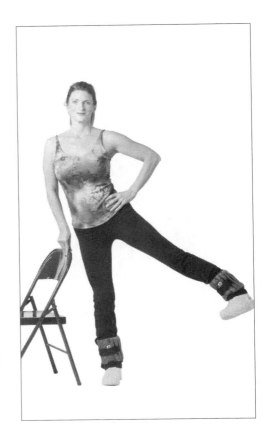

Exercise Technique

1. Begin with the leg that is away from the chair. Rotate the toes inward toward your body. Keeping the toes rotated inward, lead with the heel and exhale as you lift the leg directly out to the side up as far as you can comfortably go without moving your hips.

2. Lower the leg back down to start position in a controlled manner, grazing your foot onto the floor but not resting it before you lift again.

REPEAT 8 TO 12 TIMES, MOVE TO THE OTHER SIDE OF THE CHAIR, AND REPEAT WITH THE OTHER LEG.

Prone Leg Press

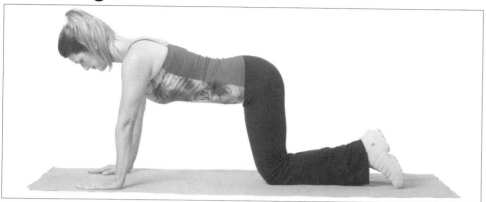

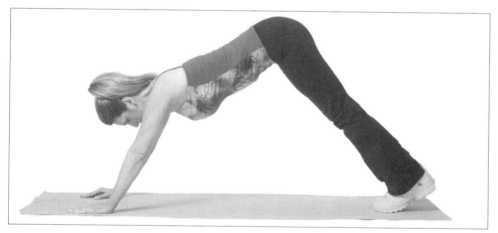

Exercise Technique

1. Exhale as you straighten your knees and tighten the front of your thighs at the top of the move.

2. Reverse the move and bend at the knees, stopping just before your knees rest back down onto the floor.

REPEAT 8 TO 12 TIMES.

BODY PART WORKED
Front of Thighs (Quadricep)

SET UP
Get on your hands and knees with the abdominal muscles held in tight. Your knees should be together and directly under your hips and your fingers should be pointing straight ahead.

TIPS FROM JONI
Be sure to maintain proper breathing during this move since the tendency can be to hold your breath.
Keep your neck in line with your spine throughout the move.

CHAPTER 7
Total Body

ROUTINE A

BODY PART WORKED

Chest (Pectoral)

SET UP

Lie on a step with your back flat and neck supported. Hold a bar in each hand and extend both arms straight up from your shoulders in line with your chest, with palms facing in forward.

TIPS FROM JONI

Keep your wrists straight throughout the move.

Chest Press On Step

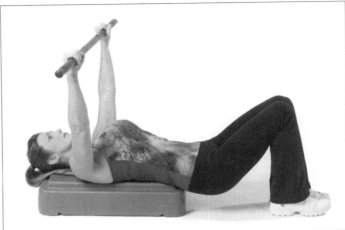

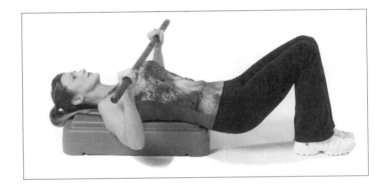

Exercise Technique

1. Bend at the elbows as you lower the weight straight downward, stopping when you feel a stretch through the chest.

2. Exhale as you extend your arms, pressing the weight straight back up to start position.

REPEAT 8 TO 12 TIMES.

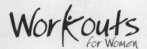

Pulse Up Crunches

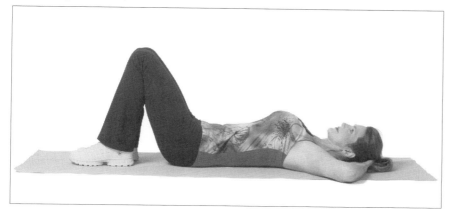

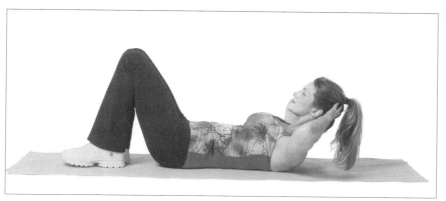

BODY PART WORKED
Upper Abdomen (Rectus Abdominis)

SET UP
Lie flat on your back with your knees bent, heels close to your body and pelvis tilted slightly upward to help flatten the back. Place your fingertips lightly on the back of your head.

TIPS FROM JONI
Keep your elbows back and out of sight.
Focus your eyes upward and keep your chin one fist distance off your chest at all times.

Exercise Technique
1. Exhale and lift your shoulder blades up and forward while contracting your abdominal muscles in a pulsing up–and–down motion without allowing your head to rest back down in between pulses.

REPEAT UNTIL FATIGUED.

CHAPTER 7
Total Body

ROUTINE B

BODY PART WORKED

Hips and Buttocks, Inner and Outer Thigh (Gluteus Maximus, Adductor, Abductor)

SET UP

Grip a bar with palms facing forward and carefully raise it over your head, bringing it down to rest on top of your shoulders behind your neck. Stand straight with feet together and abdominal muscles held in tight, shoulders back, chest high and toes pointing straight ahead.

TIPS FROM JONI

Be careful not to lock your knees as you return to start position. As you lower, be sure that your knees stay directly over your ankles and do not move past your toes. Keep your elbows rotated forward throughout the move to assist in keeping proper posture. As you return to your standing position between each step, press up through your heels.

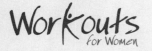

Weighted Crabs

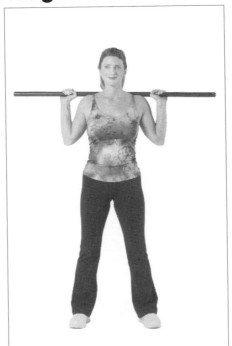
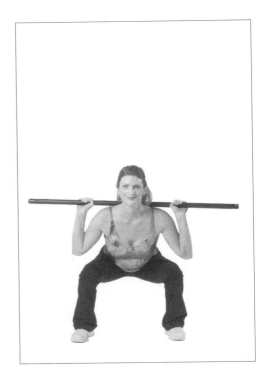

Exercise Technique

1. Begin this exercise by bending at the knees as you step out directly to the side with one leg, reaching back with your buttocks as if you were sitting back onto a chair behind you.

2. Stop when your hips are knee level. Do not drop any lower.

3. Exhale as you press yourself back up to standing position by bringing the leg that was stationary in toward the direction of the leg that had first stepped out to the side.

4. Contract the buttocks at the top of the move as you stand back up.

TAKE 10 SQUATTING STEPS IN ONE DIRECTION. REPEAT WITH THE OTHER LEG IN THE OPPOSITE DIRECTION.

Single Bicep Curl

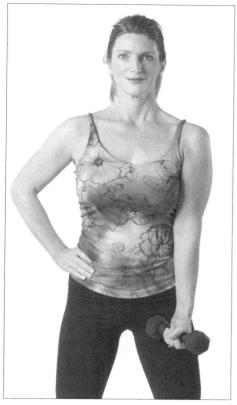 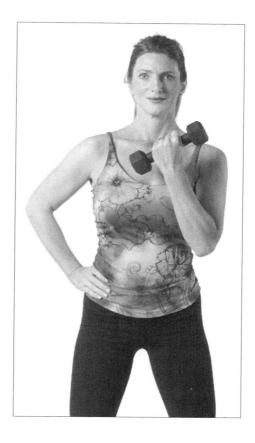

BODY PART WORKED
Front of Arms (Bicep)

SET UP
Stand tall with your shoulders back, chest out and abdominal muscles held in tight. Hold a dumbbell in one hand and rest your elbow against your hip. Extend your arm straight down, ending with the palm of your hand facing out.

TIPS FROM JONI
Be sure not to lock your elbow when lowering your arm back down to start position. Keep elbow stationary throughout the move.

Exercise Technique

1. Exhale as you bend your arm at the elbow, bringing the hand up toward your shoulder with the palm facing in at the top of the move.

2. Extend your arm back down to start in a controlled manner.

REPEAT 8 TO 12 TIMES ON ONE SIDE, THEN ON THE OTHER.

CHAPTER 7
Total Body

ROUTINE B

BODY PART WORKED

Hips and Thighs (Adductor, Abductor, Quadricep)

SET UP

Place a step in front of you with the long side facing you. Stand up straight behind your step with shoulders back, chest high, abdominal muscles held in tight and hands on your waist.

TIPS FROM JONI

Be careful to keep the knee of the bending leg behind the toes or you will be placing too much pressure on your knees.

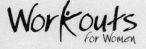

Side Lunge Touch Downs

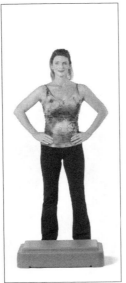 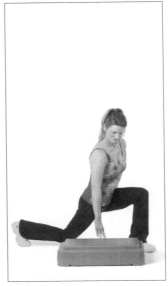 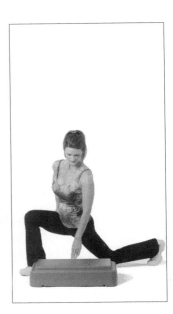

Exercise Technique

1. Extend one leg out to the side while simultaneously bending the opposite knee as you touch down onto the step with the hand on the same side as the extended leg.

2. Exhale as you pull your extended leg back in and push yourself up with the heel of the other leg. Then repeat the move on the other side.

ALTERNATE RIGHT AND LEFT FOR A TOTAL OF 16 TO 20 TIMES.

Wide Grip Push-Ups

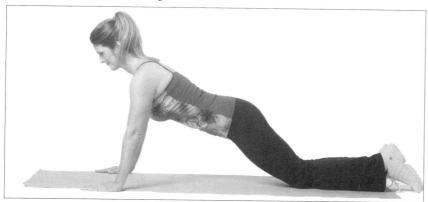

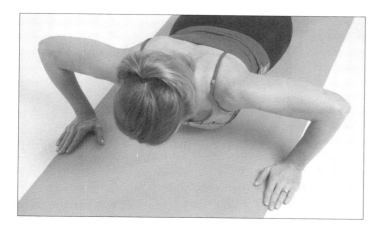

Exercise Technique

1. Bend your elbows and lower your chest, stopping one fist distance from the floor.

2. Exhale as you push your body back up to start position again.

REPEAT 8 TO 12 TIMES.

BODY PART WORKED
Chest (Pectoral)

SET UP
Get on your hands and knees with hands placed outside shoulder width, fingers facing forward and knees extended back as far as comfortable. Hold your abdominal muscles in tight.

TIPS FROM JONI
Keep elbows soft (slightly bent) as you extend back up to start position. Keep abdominal muscles tight and your neck in line with your spine at all times. To decrease the difficulty of the move, bring your hands and knees in closer together.

CHAPTER 7
Total Body

ROUTINE B

BODY PART WORKED

Mid-Back (Latissimus Dorsi, Rhomboid)

SET UP

Begin this exercise in a semi-lunge position, standing with one leg forward and one back. Both knees should be pointing straight ahead and abdominal muscles should be held in tight. Lean forward, bending at the hip, and rest the forward hand on your forward thigh to support your body. Hold a dumbbell in the other hand and position the arm hanging down holding the weight near the forward knee.

TIPS FROM JONI

Be sure to keep your forward hand on the thigh to support your back throughout the move.

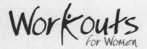

Bent Over Row To Ribs

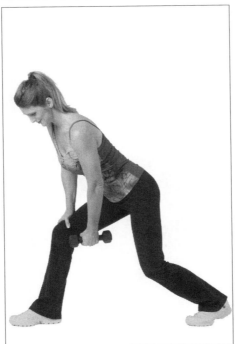
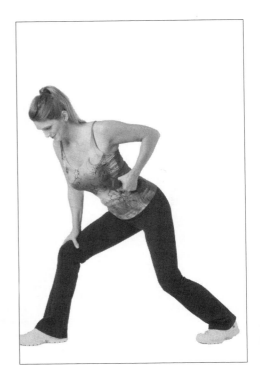

Exercise Technique

1. Keeping your hand close to your body, exhale as you lift the weight straight up toward your ribcage, squeezing the shoulder blades together at the top of the movement.

2. Lower the weight back down to start position.

REPEAT 8 TO 12 TIMES ON ONE SIDE, THEN ON THE OTHER.

Alternating Forward Raises

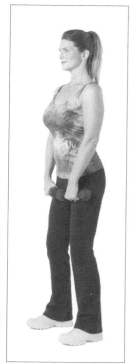 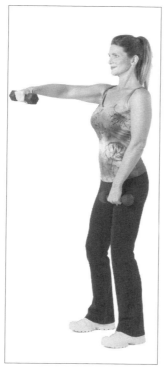 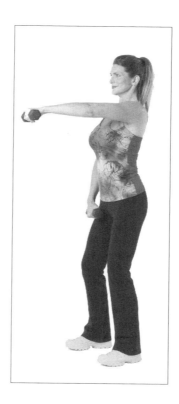

BODY PART WORKED

Front of Shoulders
(Posterior Deltoid)

SET UP

Stand tall with abdominal muscles held in tight, shoulders back and chest high. Hold a dumbbell in each hand with your palms facing in, resting on your thighs in front of your body.

TIPS FROM JONI

Keep a slight bend in your knees during this move to release some pressure from your back as you lift the weight up in front of your body.

Exercise Technique

1. Exhale as you raise up one arm directly in front of your body, stopping at shoulder height.

2. Lower arm back down in a controlled manner and repeat on the other side.

REPEAT A TOTAL OF 20 TIMES, ALTERNATING RIGHT AND LEFT.

CHAPTER 7
Total Body

ROUTINE B

BODY PART WORKED

Chest/Back of Arms
(Pectoral, Triceps)

SET UP

Get on your hands and knees with your hands directly under your shoulders and fingers facing forward. Hold your abdominal muscles in tight.

TIPS FROM JONI

Be careful not to lock your elbows as you push back up to start position. Keep your neck in line with your spine throughout the move.

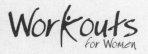

Triceps Push Ups

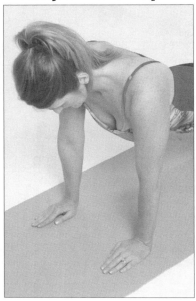

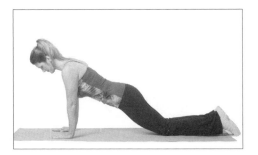

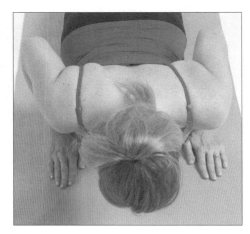

Exercise Technique

1. Bend at the elbows and lower your chest, stopping one fist distance from the floor.

2. Exhale as you push back up to start position, straightening your arms.

REPEAT 8 TO 12 TIMES.

Mule Pulses

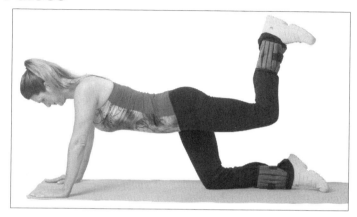

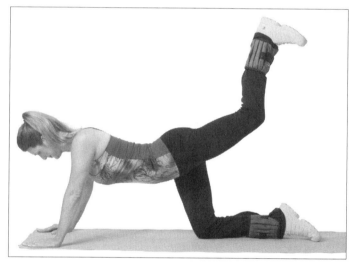

Exercise Technique

1. Pulse (tiny upward movement) the leg up by squeezing the buttocks at the top of the move.

REPEAT 8 TO 12 TIMES ON ONE SIDE, THEN 15 ON THE OTHER.

ROUTINE B

BODY PART WORKED
Buttocks (Gluteus Maximus)

SET UP
With ankle weights around each leg, get onto your knees and forearms. Lift up one leg, keeping a 90 degree angle at the knee with the foot flexed.

TIPS FROM JONI
Keep your neck in a relaxed position.
Keep both hips square to the ground during the entire movement.

CHAPTER 7
Total Body

ROUTINE B

BODY PART WORKED

Outer Thigh (Abductor)

SET UP

Lie on your side with the top arm supporting the weight in front of your body. Hips and legs should be directly on top of each other and knees should be bent at a 90 degree angle. Hold abdominal muscles in tight.

TIPS FROM JONI

Be sure to keep your hips stacked directly on top of each other for maximum effectiveness.

Bent Outer Thigh

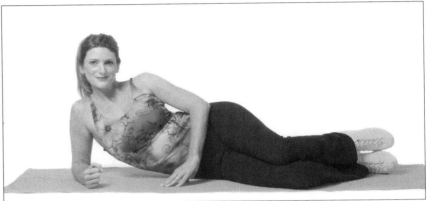

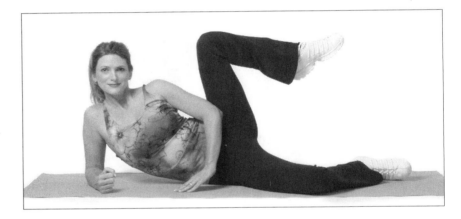

Exercise Technique

1. Exhale as you lift the top leg as high as you can, keeping your knee bent and motionless.

2. Control the leg as you lower back to start without resting the leg.

REPEAT 8 TO 12 TIMES ON ONE SIDE, THEN REPEAT ON THE OPPOSITE.

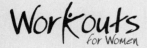

Reverse Bicycle Crunch

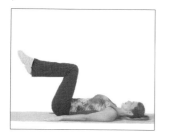 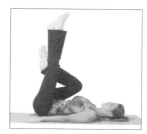 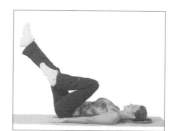

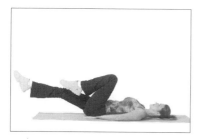 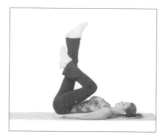

BODY PART WORKED

Lower Abdomen (Rectus Abdominis)

SET UP

Lie flat on your back with both legs lifted up with knees bent and together. Place your hands at your sides with palms facing down.

TIPS FROM JONI

Lifting up with the pelvis is what creates the focus on your abdominal muscles. Be sure not to initiate the lift by using rocking and momentum.

Exercise Technique

1. Exhale as you extend one leg straight up as you simultaneously lift the pelvis.

2. Now lower the leg and the pelvis, bringing the knee in toward the chest. When you are midway back to start position, begin to extend the other leg straight up as you simultaneously lift the pelvis.

ALTERNATE RIGHT AND LEFT UNTIL FATIGUED.

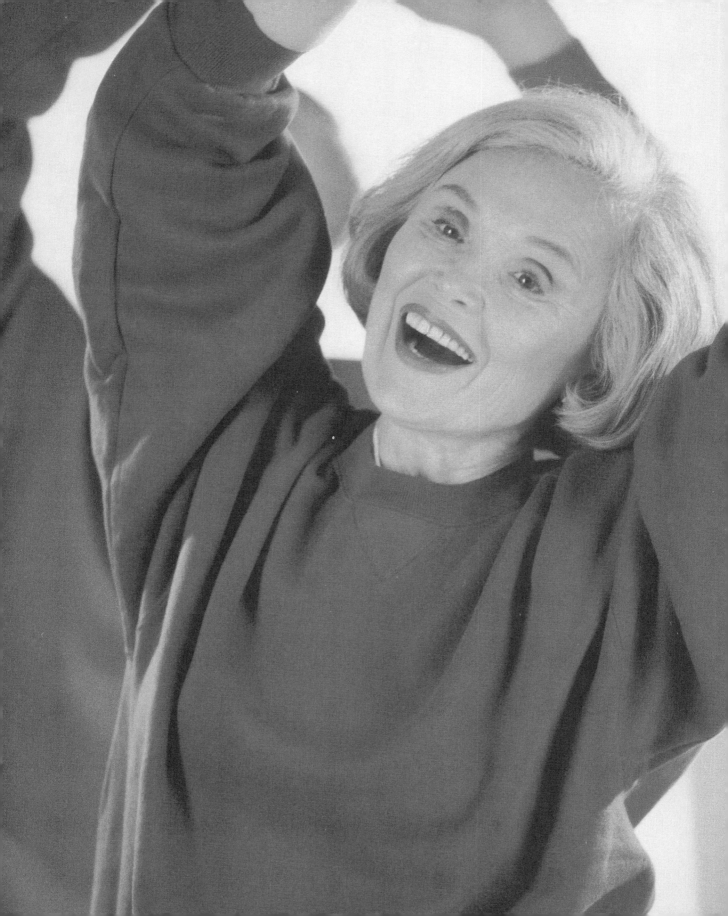

CHAPTER 8

Stretch Routine

Stretching at the end of your workout is the most effective way to produce permanent gains in flexibility since the muscles and ligament temperature are slightly elevated. Furthermore, stretching can offer mental and physical relaxation after a workout. So, stretching is highly recommended at the end of your workout. Here are some key points to remember when stretching:

1. Proper stretching is critical in achieving maximum benefits and preventing injury. Follow instructions as written and as shown in the photographs.

2. Slowly lengthen the muscle in a controlled manner to the point where you feel slight discomfort.

3. Hold that position for 15 to 30 seconds.

4. Do not bounce or jerk; HOLD.

The benefits of stretching include reduced risk for injury to muscles, joints and tendons, reduction in muscular soreness and tension and the increased ability to perform movements, including everyday functions.

Kneeling Child's Pose Shoulder Stretch

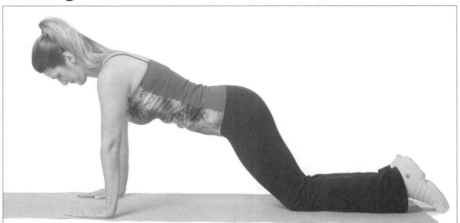

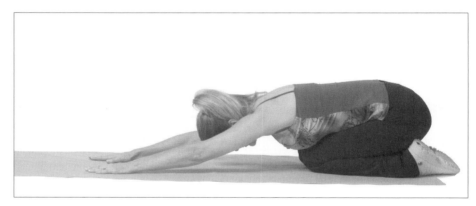

Exercise Technique

1. Exhale as you sit back, moving your buttocks toward your heels while extending your arms out in front of your body. Keep your elbows straight and palms facing down. Allow your head and neck to relax.

2. Extend until you feel mild tension through the shoulder areas.

HOLD FOR 30 SECONDS.

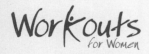

Lying Torso Twist

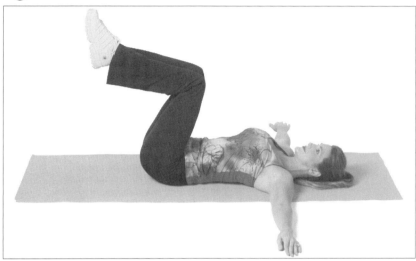

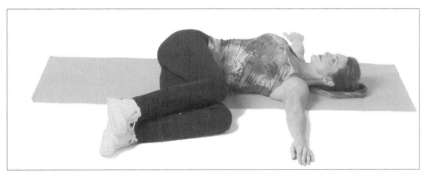

MUSCLES STRETCHED
Erector Spinae

SET UP
Lie on your back with both knees bent and feet flat on the floor.

Exercise Technique

1. Keeping your feet and knees together, lift your feet off the floor so your lower legs are parallel to the floor.

2. Keeping knees together, exhale and carefully rotate the torso to the side until the lower leg is now resting on the floor, with the opposite leg stacked directly on top.

3. Keep your shoulder blades on the floor and go to the point at which you feel mild tension in your lower back.

HOLD FOR 30 SECONDS.

CHAPTER 8
Stretch Routine

SET UP

Sit tall on the floor with your knees bent and the bottom of your feet together.

Inner Thigh Stretch

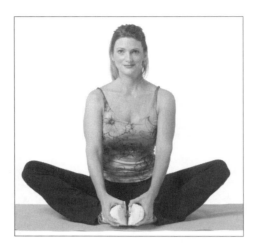 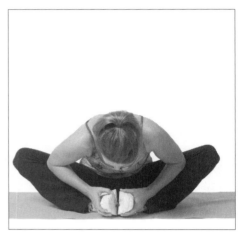

Exercise Technique

1. Bring your feet in toward your body.

2. Grasp your feet and exhale as you lean your chest forward, gently pressing downward with your forearms onto your thighs.

3. Extend until you feel mild tension in your inner thighs.

HOLD FOR 30 SECONDS.

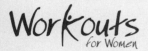

Back of Leg Stretch

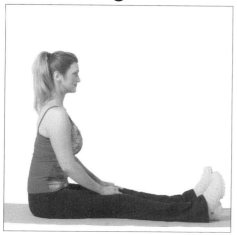 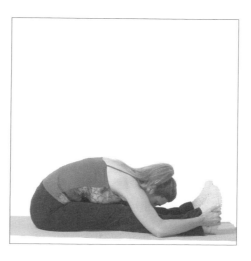

SET UP

Sit tall with both legs extended straight out in front of you about shoulder width apart.

Exercise Technique

1. Exhale as you bend forward at the hips and reach toward your ankles.

2. Extend until you feel mild tension in the back of the legs.

HOLD FOR 30 SECONDS.

SET UP

Get on your hands and
knees.

Prone Hip and Buttocks Stretch

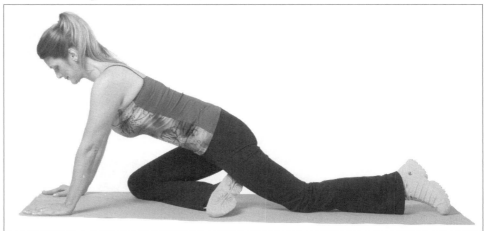

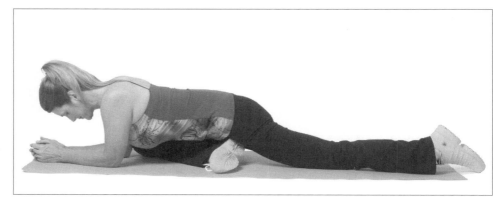

Exercise Technique

1. Slide the right knee forward. Now angle your leg so that the right foot
    crosses over to the left side of your body.

2. Slide the left leg straight back. Your instep should be facing down with the
    left leg extended straight out. Your right foot should now be under your left
    hip.

3. Exhale as you lower your upper body down so that you are resting on your
    forearms.

4. Extend until you feel mild tension in the hip and buttocks area.

HOLD FOR 30 SECONDS.

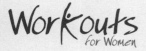

Chest Stretch

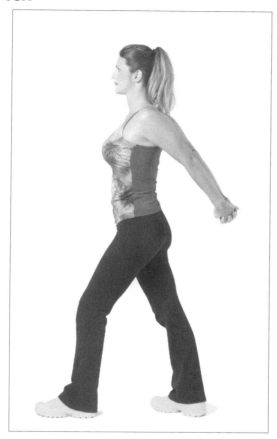

MUSCLES STRETCHED
Pectoral

SET UP
Stand tall and reach arms behind you, interlocking the fingers if your flexibility will allow.

Exercise Technique

1. Exhale as you pull your shoulder blades together and down while lifting your chest upward.

2. Extend until you feel mild tension through the chest.

HOLD FOR 30 SECONDS.

MUSCLES STRETCHED

Triceps

SET UP

Stand tall. Drop your chin down toward your chest.

Back of Arms Stretch

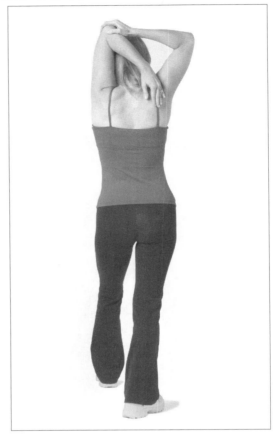

Exercise Technique

1. Reach one arm straight up overhead with the palm of your hand facing for-ward.

2. Bend your arm at the elbow and drop your hand to the back of your neck with your palm facing in.

3. Exhale as you reach overhead with the opposite arm and grasp the other arm just below the elbow.

4. Gently pull the other arm in toward the center of your head.

5. Extend until you feel mild tension in the back of the upper arm.

HOLD FOR 30 SECONDS, THEN REPEAT ON THE OTHER SIDE.

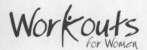

Standing Thigh Stretch

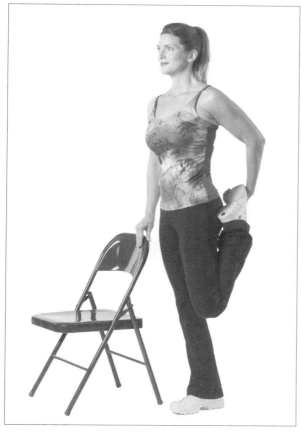

SET UP

Stand tall, holding onto a wall or chair for balance.

Exercise Technique

1. Bend your right knee up behind you as you reach back and grasp the right ankle with the right hand, pulling the heel toward your buttocks.

2. Exhale as you gently draw your heel up and in toward your buttocks.

3. Extend until you feel mild tension in the front of your thigh.

HOLD FOR 30 SECONDS, THEN REPEAT ON THE OTHER SIDE. BE CAREFUL NOT TO OVERSTRETCH THE KNEE.

Calf Stretch

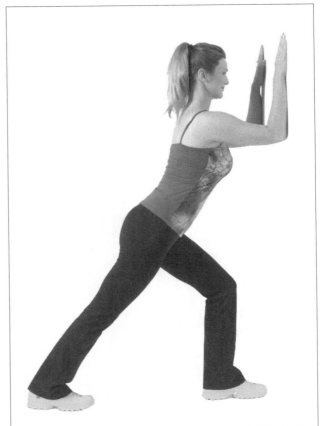

Exercise Technique

1. Place your forearms against the wall and lean forward.

2. Exhale as you step back with one leg and press the heel down.

3. Extend until you feel mild tension in the lower rear area of the extended leg.

HOLD FOR 30 SECONDS.

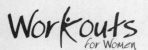

Standing Abdomen and Back Stretch

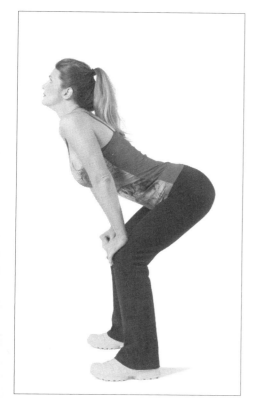 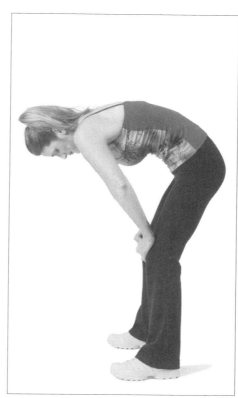

MUSCLES STRETCHED
Rectus Abdominis, Erector Spinae

SET UP
Stand with feet shoulder width apart.

Exercise Technique

1. Bend forward at the hips and rest hands just above your knees with your fingers pointing in toward each other.

2. Exhale as you tuck your chin in toward your chest as you round back upward, feeling mild tension through the back.

HOLD FOR 10 SECONDS.

3. Release the hold and exhale as you reverse the arch in the back to a downward arch by lifting your head and tail bone up, now feeling mild tension through the back.

HOLD FOR 10 SECONDS. ALTERNATE BETWEEN THE TWO POSITIONS, 2 TO 4 TIMES EACH.

SET UP

Stand with your abdominal muscles held in tight, shoulders back and chest high. Point your toes and knees straight ahead.

Neck Rolls

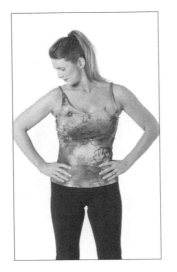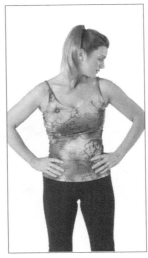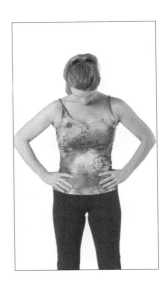

Exercise Technique

1. Exhale as you drop your chin toward your chest.

2. Keeping your chin close to your body, gently roll your neck from shoulder to shoulder in a smooth, controlled motion.

REPEAT THIS SIDE-TO-SIDE ROLLING MOTION 5 TIMES.

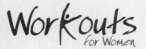

Standing Torso Stretch

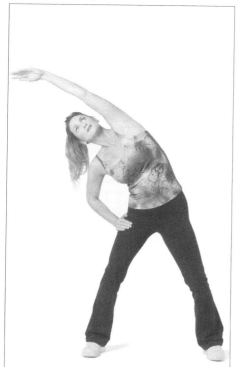 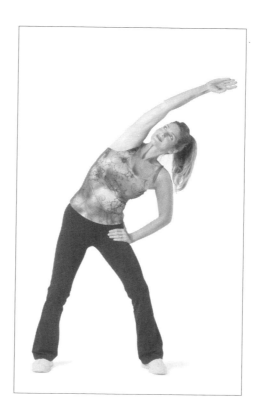

SET UP

Stand with your abdominal muscles held in tight, shoulders back and chest high with legs double shoulder width apart. Point your toes and knees straight ahead.

Exercise Technique

1. Place one hand on the corresponding hip for support.

2. Exhale while you reach overhead with the opposite arm, bending your torso in the opposite direction.

3. Extend until you feel mild tension through the side of your torso.

HOLD FOR 30 SECONDS, THEN REPEAT ON THE OTHER SIDE.

Part
3

Putting It Together

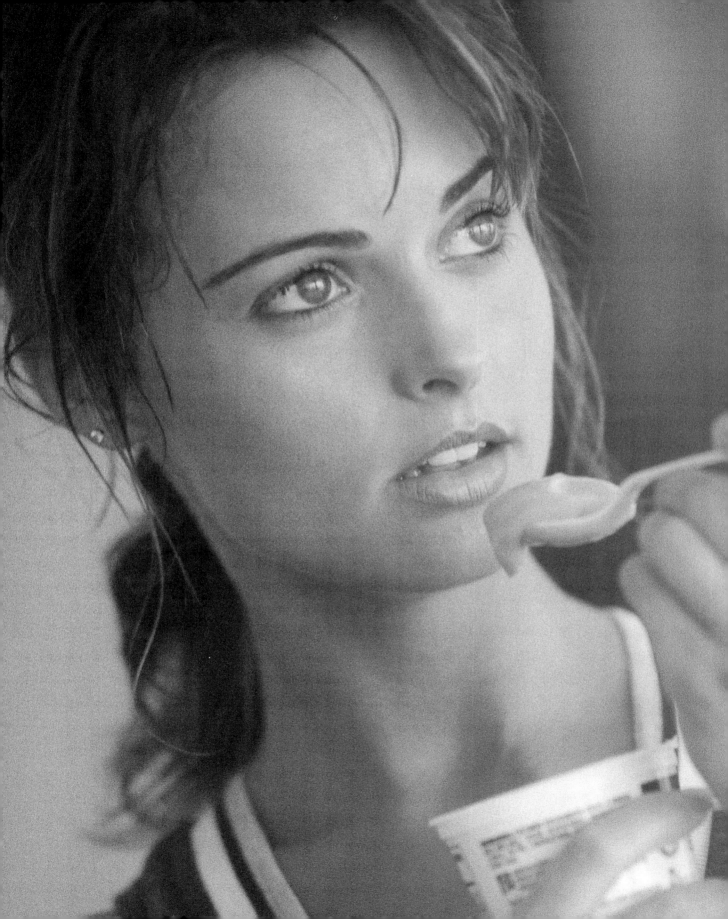

Nutrition: Clear and Simple

Fitness and Nutrition — A Successful Combination!

You have chosen a Workouts for Women fitness program, but a good physical fitness regimen is only part of the equation. Ongoing exercise and healthy eating habits contribute to a balanced lifestyle and this combination is crucial in achieving long-term results. You will need to constantly renew that commitment to a better, healthier life with your everyday decisions. The fitness and nutrition partnership will lead to success!

Understanding the New USDA Food Guide Pyramid and 2005 Dietary Guidelines for Americans

The American public continues to become better educated regarding fitness and nutritional information. Consequently, the government and private institutions are involved in ongoing research programs to elicit the most accurate data. The USDA recently revised the Food Guide Pyramid and provided more detailed information in easier-to-understand terminology. The new pyramid stresses a combination of exercise and nutritious foods while highlighting the concept that without both, an individual will not be able to achieve long-term weight control and optimal health.

General food guidelines for nutritious eating as recommended by the USDA 2005 Dietary Guidelines for Americans are as follows:

- Grains: At least half of all the grains that you consume should be whole grains, including whole-wheat flour, oatmeal, popcorn and cereals.
- Vegetables: Eat more dark green and orange vegetables. Try crunchy vegetables that are raw or steamed. Also, drink 100 percent vegetable juices.
- Fruit: Drink fruit juice in moderation. Opt for a wide variety of fresh, canned, frozen or dried fruit.
- Dairy: The USDA recommends three cups of low-fat or fat-free milk, yogurt and cheese daily.

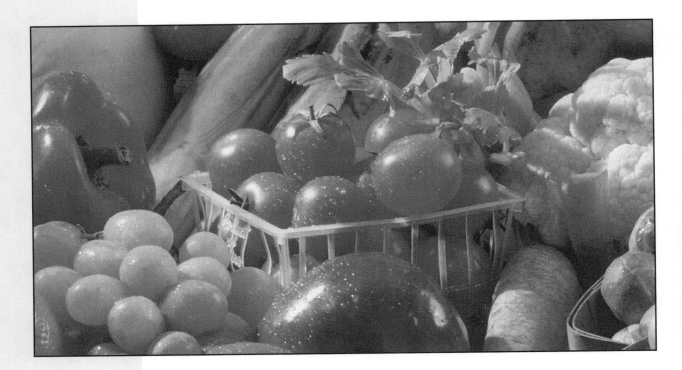

- Meat and Beans: This group includes meat, poultry, fish, dry beans, peas, eggs, nuts, and seeds. Opt for low-fat or lean meats and poultry that can be baked, broiled or grilled. Fish, nuts, and seeds contain healthy oils. Choose these items frequently in place of meats or poultry.
- Fats: Most of the fat in your diet should come from fish, nuts, and vegetable oils. Limit solid fats such as butter, stick margarine, shortening, and lard.

Visit www.mypyramid.gov for the USDA's new personalized approach to healthy eating.

Mini Meals Are Part of the Solution

Research has shown that eating five or six smaller meals (Mini Meals) each day has substantial benefits as opposed to the traditional, larger three square meals per day. As a result, the first step toward weight loss and subsequent long-term weight control is the adoption of a smaller Mini Meal pattern. A healthy Mini Meal consists of 150 to 400 calories and contains a balance of carbohydrates, fats and protein.

Three main benefits of a Mini Meal plan are:

1. Your body will burn up to 10 percent more calories per day due to the "thermal effect." When you eat smaller meals more often versus the fewer, but larger, square meals, your body maintains a higher metabolism and is able to burn off more calories.

2. Lower stress is placed on your heart. Eating a large meal increases an individual's risk of having a heart attack by causing the heart to beat up to 30 percent faster. Smaller meals reduce this effect.

3. Blood sugar levels remain stabilized with frequent Mini Meals. Insulin surges that occur during the time lapses between three large meals can be prevented, thereby decreasing unhealthy cravings, mood swings, and headaches.

Three-Day Mini Meal Plan

IMPORTANT: This meal plan is designed to promote weight loss in healthy individuals. This advice should not replace or take precedence over the advice of your health care provider. Please consult with your health care provider before beginning this meal plan and follow his or her recommendation.

Healthy eating and exercise go hand in hand. To maximize your energy level while excercising and to ensure that your metabolism is running efficiently, proper nutrition through balanced meals is essential. This three-day meal plan features the following:

- carbohydrates with low to moderate glycemic index values to raise blood sugar levels gradually, reducing the production of the fat-storing hormone insulin
- five small meals every day, which research has shown to be healthier and more beneficial than the traditional three larger meals
- Mini Meals that are approximately 400 calories, with snacks at approximately 150 calories to maintain a caloric intake of 1,500 calories per day
- small frequent meals that are high in fiber to promote weight loss, lower cholesterol levels and stabilize blood sugar levels
- Mini Meals that include a variety of fresh produce and herbs creating meals high in phytonutrients; key to maintaining optimal health
- Mini Meals that emphasize a diet low in processed foods and refined sugars. Included are whole grains and plentiful servings of fresh fruits, vegetables and high biological value proteins to maximize the amount of nutrients per meal
- evenly spaced meals throughout the day to keep your appetite satisfied

Mini Meal Plan Options

Breakfast

VANILLA PEANUT BUTTER YOGURT CRUNCH
1 cup (8 oz.) non-fat vanilla yogurt
1/4 cup low-fat granola
1/8 cup Grape-Nuts Cereal
1 T. crunchy peanut butter

Mix granola, cereal and peanut butter with the yogurt.

FRIED EGGS WITH SWEET POTATO HOME FRIES
2 large eggs, fried
1 medium sweet potato, baked, peeled, and sliced/chopped
1 pink/red Florida grapefruit, cut in half

Coat nonstick skillet with cooling spray and place on medium-high heat. Add baked sweet potato pieces and fry until browned. Serve with fried eggs.

CRUNCHY ALMOND COTTAGE CHEESE WITH TANGERINE SLICES
1 1/2 cups low-fat cottage cheese
1 medium tangerine
3 T. almond slices

Combine nuts and tangerine slices with cottage cheese.

Morning Snack

APPLE AND PEANUTS
1/2 medium apple
1/8 cup dry roasted peanuts, unsalted

YOGURT COVERED RAISINS WITH DRY ROASTED PEANUTS
1/8 cup yogurt-covered raisins
1/16 cup dry roasted peanuts, unsalted

Combine yogurt-covered raisins and peanuts.

CARROT RAISIN SALAD
1 cup grated carrots
1 minibox (0.5 oz.) seedless raisins
1 T. light mayonnaise

Stir all ingredients in a bowl.

Lunch

TURKEY SANDWICH
2 oz. deli sliced turkey
1 oz. Swiss cheese
2 slices pumpernickel bread, whole grain
2 (1/4" thick) slice fresh tomato
1 large slice red onion
2 pieces inner leaf romaine lettuce
1 T. light mayonnaise
1 T. brown mustard

Spread mayonnaise and mustard on each bread slice and layer all ingredients in between.

TUNA SANDWICH
4 oz. canned solid white tuna in water
2 T. light mayonnaise
2 T. red onion, chopped
2 T. celery, chopped
1 (1/4" thick) slice fresh tomato
3 fresh spinach leaves
2 slices pumpernickel bread, whole grain

Mix canned tuna with mayo, celery and onion. Toast bread (optional). Scoop tuna on top of bread. Top with spinach leaves and tomato and second slice of bread.

GRILLED CHICKEN CAESAR WRAP
4 oz. cubed grilled chicken breast
1/2 cup romaine lettuce, chopped
2 T. Parmesan cheese, grated
2 T. low calorie caesar salad dressing
1 whole-wheat tortilla (7-8")

Mix all ingredients. Add to warm tortilla and roll.

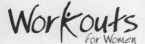

Afternoon Snack

HUMMUS OVER WARMED PITA

1/2 whole-wheat pita (6 1/2")
3 T. hummus

Warm or toast pita and cut into 3 slices. Spread 1 T. hummus on each slice.

CHEESY SPINACH

2 cups baby spinach
2 T. part-skim mozzarella cheese, grated
2 T. Parmesan cheese, grated
1 tsp. canola oil

Steam spinach. While hot, mix with canola oil and sprinkle with cheese. Microwave for 20 seconds if necessary to melt cheese.

COOL KIWI

2 kiwi, peeled
3 T. Cool Whip Lite

Slice kiwis and top with Cool Whip.

Dinner

MEDITERRANEAN TUNA SALAD

1 (5 oz.) can solid white tuna, in water
1 cup romaine lettuce, chopped
6 red cherry tomatoes
1/4 cup feta cheese, crumbled
4 T. light Italian salad dressing

Toss vegetables, feta cheese, and salad dressing. Drain tuna and place on top.

SMOKED SALMON GORGONZOLA SALAD

6 oz. smoked salmon
2 cups romaine lettuce, chopped
2 large slices red onion
4 slices tomato, halved
10 slices cucumber, peeled and halved
2 T. Gorgonzola cheese, crumbled
2 T. capers
3 T. olive oil vinaigrette dressing

Heat salmon for 20 to 30 minutes at 400 degrees F. Prepare salad. Add salmon and top salad with Gorgonzola cheese and dressing.

CURRIED CHICKEN WITH BROWN RICE

5 oz. roasted chicken breast, boneless and skinless
1/2 cup whole-grain brown rice, cooked
1/4 stewed tomatoes, canned
2 T. golden seedless raisins
1 tsp curry powder
2 T. green onion, chopped

Put chicken in a sauté pan with tomatoes, raisins, onions, and curry powder. Bring to a simmer and cook, stirring until chicken is tender, about 10 minutes. Raise heat to bring to a boil, then simmer uncovered an additional 10 minutes. Serve over rice.

CHAPTER 9
Nutrition: Clear and Simple

Food Journals Show Results

If you are trying to lose weight and adopt healthier eating patterns, keeping track of what you eat by using a food journal can help significantly. A food journal can be a real eye-opener and can help you figure out what changes in your diet to focus on. Researchers at the Chicago Center for Behavioral Medicine & Sport Psychology say that keeping a food journal allows people to see patterns in their eating. If you have to write it down, you may think twice before having that extra cookie. Individuals who keep a journal to consistently monitor their food intake steadily lose more weight (1 to 2 pounds per week) and keep it off. Journals work for several reasons, such as:

1. By keeping a visual record of what you eat, sources of unnecessary additional calories can be identified.

2. By tracking activity patterns at meal and snack times, certain situations emerge that prompt you to overindulge in diet-destructive behavior.

3. Optimal success is measured by your personal goals. It is extremely helpful to have those goals in writing and encouraging to track your successes (or areas for improvement) daily.

Remember to keep the journal simple and to total up at the end of the day. To get started, please refer to Appendix B where you will find a blank food journal.

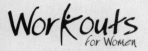

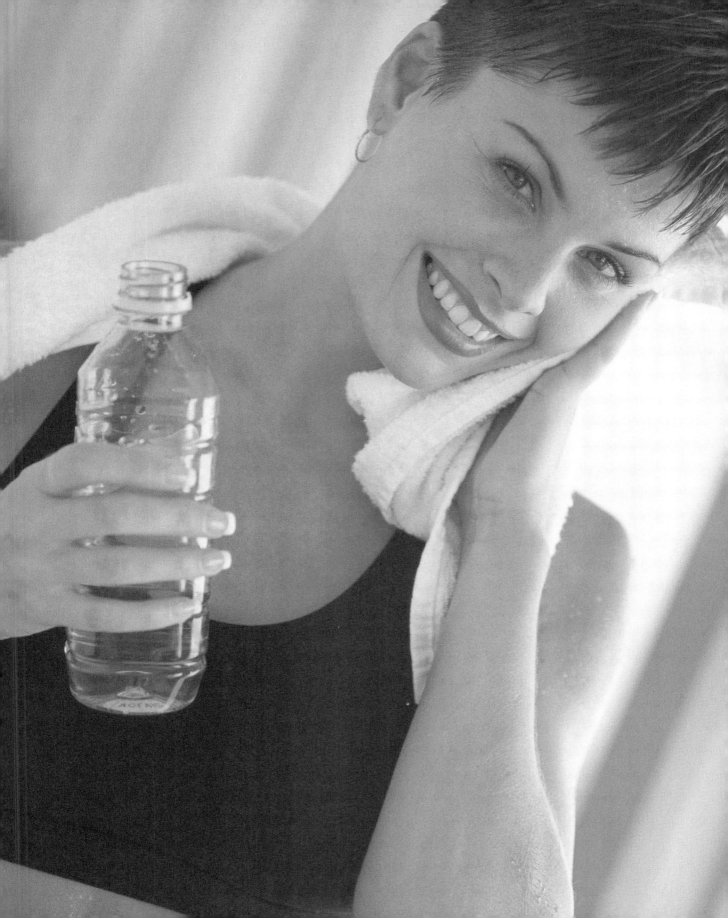

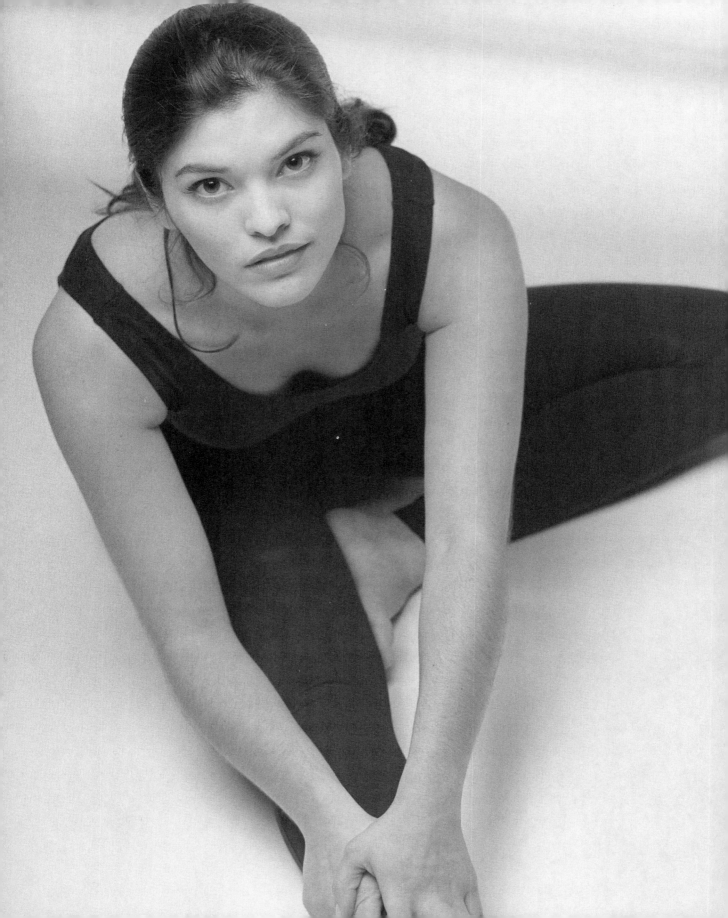

Creating a Workout

As You Progress

Remember, if you want to continue to see results over time, it is important not to let your body become too comfortable with your workouts. Keep rotating through the various scheduling options to prevent plateaus. If you find that the weight you are using for a particular exercise is no longer challenging, it is time to increase the weight. Slowly add weight without compromising form.

Note: Perform three sets of each exercise before moving on to the next exercise. Aerobic activity can be included on alternate days if desired, rather than completing the exercise on the same day as the weight training workouts.

A Word About Aerobic Exercise

The word "aerobic" means requiring oxygen and regarding physical activity it is defined by exercise that causes a sustained, increased heart rate. Recommended aerobic exercise duration is offered in the individual workout. The mode of aerobic activity is entirely up to you. Whether you choose biking, jogging, swimming, rowing, skating, the treadmill, or the elliptical trainer, the main thing is that you increase your heart rate for the maximum period of time during your workout.

The amount of aerobic exercise in addition to your weight training will vary depending on the amount of time you have and your goals. If you are trying to lose weight quickly, the recommendation is 30 minutes of aerobic exercise, 5 days per week in addition to one of the weight training workout schedules. Avoid being too aggressive with your workout schedule so that you do not burn out and quit. For a more moderate pace, complete three 30-minute aerobic sessions per week in addition to one of the weight training schedules.

Zone Workouts Schedule

To maximize specific muscular results, your body has been divided into five different Zones:

1. Shoulders and Arms

2. Chest and Back

3. Lower Body

4. Abdominals and Lower Back

5. Total Body

Two completely different exercise routines (routine A and B) are offered for each Zone to mix it up a little while still focusing on your targeted body area. Each daily workout consists of the different Zones you have selected and the exercise group you have chosen. Four-week rotating Zone Workout schedules are offered in a 3-, 4-, or 5- day format with coordinated aerobic exercise recommendations. Obviously, the 4- and 5-day plans will show results faster, but a 3-day plan is perfect if you prefer to reach your goals at a moderate pace, or for a maintenance program.

All of the workouts are appropriate for women who are just beginning their fitness program and for women who are experienced trainers. Just follow the guidelines to adapt weight and sets to your level. So, create your flexible plan by deciding what Zones to target, picking the Zone exercise group and selecting the day format.

Personalize Your Workout

Each day, you are given different zones to exercise. It's up to you whether you would like to perform Routine A or B from that Zone. This is designed to give you some variation in your workout and to make sure your exercise stays fresh, new, and different. Both are designed at the same stress level, so you may switch from A to B without worrying about an increase or decrease in difficulty.

You are the one that must be the judge of how your body reacts to the workouts. The workouts call for 3 sets of 8 to 12 repetitions for each exercise, and a rest of 30 seconds at the end of each set. However, your body may have to build up to this point. If you find that you are unable to finish the Zone, try cutting back the number of sets you perform to 2. If at any point you find yourself unable to perform an exercise with proper form, stop! You are here to workout and tone your body, not to potentially injure yourself.

Remember, have fun and get ready to work out!

Workouts for Women

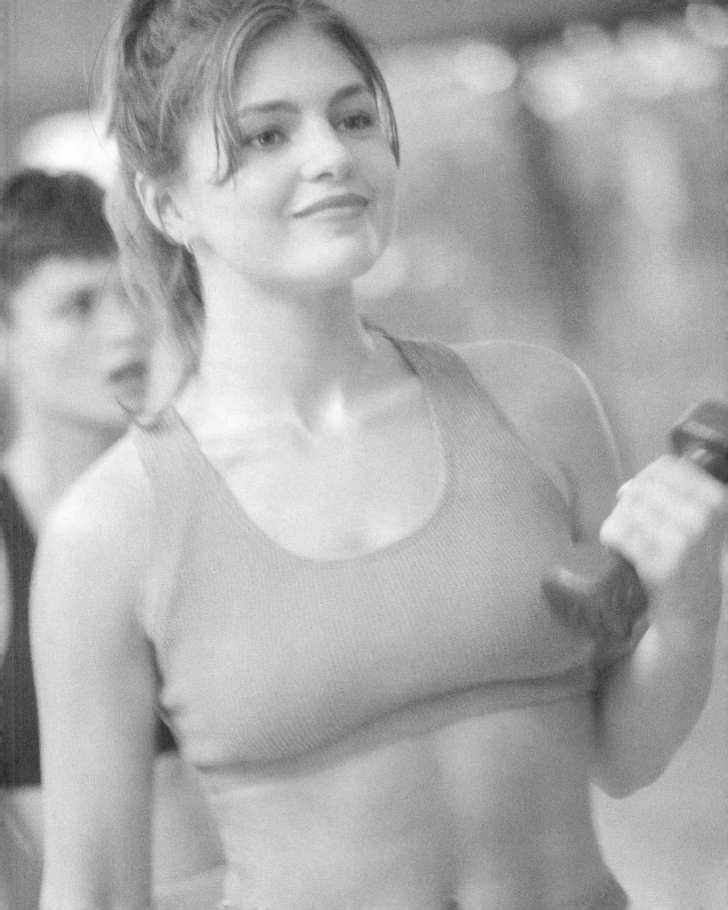

3 Day Week 1

Sunday
Shoulders and Arms — page 18
Lower Body — page 42

Monday
Rest Day

Tuesday
Chest and Back — page 30
Abdominals and
   Lower Back — page 55
Aerobic Activity

Wednesday
Rest Day

Thursday
Total Body — page 68
Aerobic Activity

Friday
Rest Day

Saturday
Rest Day

3 Day Week 2

Sunday
Lower Body — page 42
Chest and Back — page 30

Monday
Rest Day

Tuesday
Shoulders and Arms — page 18
Abdominals and
   Lower Back — page 55
Aerobic Activity

Wednesday
Rest Day

Thursday
Lower Body — page 42
Abdominals and
   Lower Back — page 55
Aerobic Activity

Friday
Rest Day

Saturday
Rest Day

Workouts for Women

3 Day Week 3

Sunday
Total Body   page 68

Monday
Rest Day

Tuesday
Shoulders and Arms   page 18
Lower Body   page 42
Aerobic Activity

Wednesday
Rest Day

Thursday
Lower Body   page 42
Abdominals and
   Lower Back   page 55
Aerobic Activity

Friday
Rest Day

Saturday
Rest Day

3 Day Week 4

Sunday
Lower Body   page 42
Chest and Back   page 30

Monday
Rest Day

Tuesday
Total Body   page 42
Aerobic Activity

Wednesday
Rest Day

Thursday
Shoulders and Arms   page 18
Abdominals and
   Lower Back   page 55
Aerobic Activity

Friday
Rest Day

Saturday
Rest Day

CHAPTER 10
Creating a Workout

117

4 Day Week 1

Sunday
Shoulders and Arms   page 18
Lower Body   page 42
Aerobic Activity

Monday
Chest and Back   page 30
Abdominals and
   Lower Back   page 55

Tuesday
Rest Day

Wednesday
Total Body   page 68
Aerobic Activity

Thursday
Shoulders and Arms   page 18
Lower Body   page 42

Friday
Rest Day

Saturday
Rest Day

4 Day Week 2

Sunday
Total Body   page 68
Aerobic Activity

Monday
Shoulders and Arms   page 18
Abdominals and
   Lower Back   page 55

Tuesday
Rest Day

Wednesday
Lower Body   page 42
Chest and Back   page 30
Aerobic Activity

Thursday
Shoulders and Arms   page 18
Abdominals and
   Lower Back   page 60

Friday
Rest Day

Saturday
Rest Day

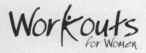

4 Day Week 3

Sunday
Shoulders and Arms   page 18
Lower Body   page 42
Aerobic Activity

Monday
Chest and Back   page 30
Abdominals and
   Lower Back   page 55

Tuesday
Rest Day

Wednesday
Total Body   page 68
Aerobic Activity

Thursday
Shoulders and Arms   page 18
Lower Body   page 42

Friday
Rest Day

Saturday
Rest Day

4 Day Week 4

Sunday
Total Body   page 68
Aerobic Activity

Monday
Shoulders and Arms   page 18
Lower Body   page 42

Tuesday
Rest Day

Wednesday
Chest and Back   page 30
Abdominals and
   Lower Back   page 55
Aerobic Activity

Thursday
Shoulders and Arms   page 18
Lower Body   page 42

Friday
Rest Day

Saturday
Rest Day

CHAPTER 10
**Creating a
Workout**

5 Day Week 1

Sunday
Shoulders and Arms	page 18
Lower Body	page 42
Aerobic Activity	

Monday
Chest and Back	page 30
Abdominals and	
Lower Back	page 55

Tuesday
Total Body	page 68
Aerobic Activity	

Wednesday
Shoulders and Arms	page 18
Abdominals and	
Lower Back	page 55

Thursday
Lower Body	page 42
Chest and Back	page 30

Friday
Rest Day

Saturday
Rest Day

5 Day Week 2

Sunday
Total Body	page 68
Aerobic Activity	

Monday
Shoulders and Arms	page 18
Abdominals and	
Lower Back	page 55

Tuesday
Lower Body	page 42
Chest and Back	page 30
Aerobic Activity	

Wednesday
Shoulders and Arms	page 18
Abdominals and	
Lower Back	page 55

Thursday
Total Body	page 68
Aerobic Activity	

Friday
Rest Day

Saturday
Rest Day

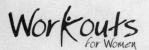

Workouts for Women

5 Day Week 3

Sunday
Lower Body	page 42
Chest and Back	page 30
Aerobic Activity	

Monday
Shoulders and Arms	page 18
Abdominals and	
Lower Back	page 55

Tuesday
Total Body	page 68
Aerobic Activity	

Wednesday
Lower Body	page 42
Abdominals and	
Lower Back	page 55

Thursday
Shoulders and Arms	page 18
Lower Body	page 42
Aerobic Activity	

Friday
Rest Day

Saturday
Rest Day

5 Day Week 4

Sunday
Lower Body	page 42
Abdominals and	
Lower Back	page 55
Aerobic Activity	

Monday
Shoulders and Arms	page 18
Chest and Back	page 30

Tuesday
Lower Body	page 42
Chest and Back	page 30
Aerobic Activity	

Wednesday
Total Body	page 68

Thursday
Shoulders and Arms	page 18
Abdominals and	
Lower Back	page 55
Aerobic Activity	

Friday
Rest Day

Saturday
Rest Day

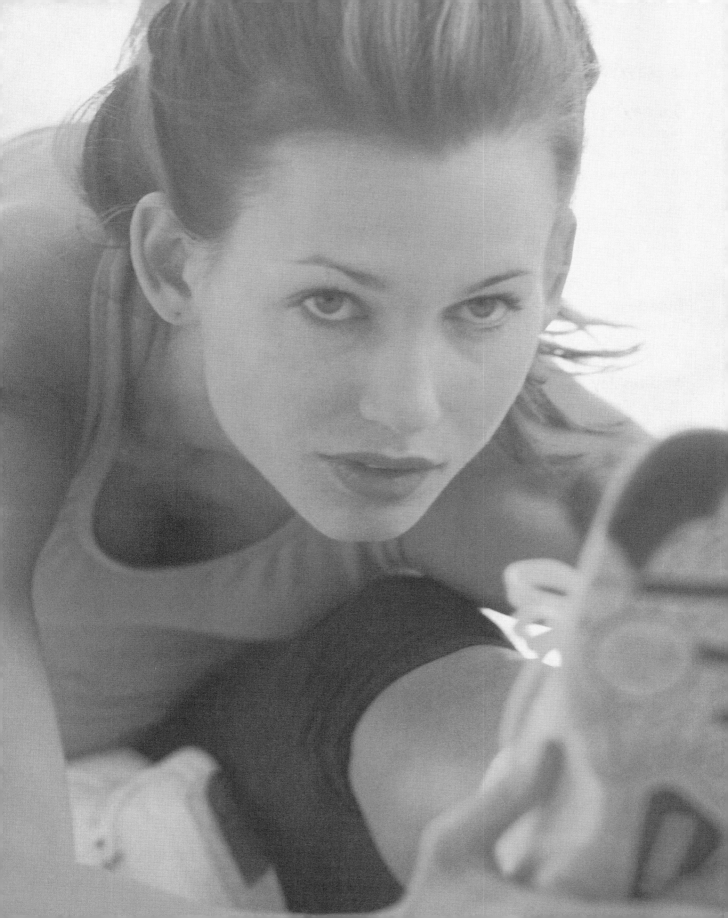

Zone/Circuit Shaping Combo Schedule

This workout puts it all together by combining Zone Training with Circuit Shaping workouts from the *Workouts for Women: Circuit Shaping* book. In addition to the Zone Workouts, Circuit Shaping exercises are incorporated into the schedule. Circuit Shaping involves a total body workout where you quickly move from one exercise to another, training various parts of the body in each session. Short intervals of aerobic activity are included for maximum calorie output. The Combo Schedule is also offered in 3-, 4-, and 5-day formats. It all adds up to maximum variety and maximum results.

Note: For more information about the *Workouts for Women: Circuit Shaping* book and video, visit us on the Web at www.WorkoutsforWomen.com.

3 Day Week 1

Sunday
Lower Body   page 42
Abdominals and
   Lower Back   page 55

Monday
Rest Day

Tuesday
Circuit 1   page 16 of *Workouts for*
Women: Circuit Training

Wednesday
Rest Day

Thursday
Shoulders and Arms   page 18
Chest and Back   page 30

Friday
Rest Day

Saturday
Rest Day

3 Day Week 2

Sunday
Lower Body   page 42
Chest and Back   page 30

Monday
Rest Day

Tuesday
Circuit 2   page 27 of *Workouts for*
Women: Circuit Training

Wednesday
Rest Day

Thursday
Shoulders and Arms   page 18
Abdominals and
   Lower Back   page 55

Friday
Rest Day

Saturday
Rest Day

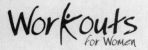

3 Day Week 3

Sunday
Shoulders and Arms	page 18
Lower Body	page 42

Monday
Rest Day

Tuesday
Circuit 3	page 38 of *Workouts for Women: Circuit Training*

Wednesday
Rest Day

Thursday
Chest and Back	page 30
Abdominals and Lower Back	page 55

Friday
Rest Day

Saturday
Rest Day

3 Day Week 4

Sunday
Lower Body	page 42
Chest and Back	page 30

Monday
Rest Day

Tuesday
Circuit 4	page 49 of *Workouts for Women: Circuit Training*

Wednesday
Rest Day

Thursday
Shoulders and Arms	page 18
Abdominals and Lower Back	page 55

Friday
Rest Day

Saturday
Rest Day

4 Day Week 1

Sunday
Lower Body   page 42

Abdominals and
   Lower Back   page 55

Monday
Circuit 5   page 60 of *Workouts for*
            Women: Circuit Training

Tuesday
Rest Day

Wednesday
Shoulders and Arms   page 18

Chest and Back   page 30

Thursday
Circuit 6   page 71 of *Workouts for*
            Women: Circuit Training

Friday
Rest Day

Saturday
Rest Day

4 Day Week 2

Sunday
Chest and Back   page 30

Abdominals and
   Lower Back   page 55

Monday
Circuit 7   page 82 of *Workouts for*
            Women: Circuit Training

Tuesday
Rest Day

Wednesday
Shoulders and Arms   page 18

Lower Body   page 42

Thursday
Circuit 8   page 94 of *Workouts for*
            Women: Circuit Training

Friday
Rest Day

Saturday
Rest Day

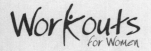

4 Day Week 3

Sunday
Shoulders and Arms   page 18
Lower Body   page 42

Monday
Circuit 9   page 105 of *Workouts for Women: Circuit Training*

Tuesday
Rest Day

Wednesday
Chest and Back   page 30
Abdominals and
    Lower Back   page 55

Thursday
Circuit 10 page 116 of *Workouts for Women: Circuit Training*

Friday
Rest Day

Saturday
Rest Day

4 Day Week 4

Sunday
Lower Body   page 42
Abdominals and
    Lower Back   page 55

Monday
Circuit 1   page 16 of *Workouts for Women: Circuit Training*

Tuesday
Rest Day

Wednesday
Shoulders and Arms   page 18
Chest and Back   page 30

Thursday
Circuit 2   page 27 of *Workouts for Women: Circuit Training*

Friday
Rest Day

Saturday
Rest Day

5 Day Week 1

Sunday
Circuit 3   page 38 of *Workouts for Women: Circuit Training*

Monday
Shoulders and Arms   page 18
Lower Body   page 42

Tuesday
Circuit 4   page 49 of *Workouts for Women: Circuit Training*

Wednesday
Chest and Back   page 30
Abdominals and
    Lower Back   page 55

Thursday
Circuit 5   page 60 of *Workouts for Women: Circuit Training*

Friday
Rest Day

Saturday
Rest Day

5 Day Week 2

Sunday
Circuit 6   page 71 of *Workouts for Women: Circuit Training*

Monday
Lower Body   page 42
Chest and Back   page 30

Tuesday
Shoulders and Arms   page 18
Abdominals and
    Lower Back   page 55

Wednesday
Lower Body   page 42
Abdominals and
    Lower Back   page 55

Thursday
Circuit 7   page 82 of *Workouts for Women: Circuit Training*

Friday
Rest Day

Saturday
Rest Day

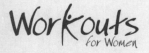

5 Day Week 3

Sunday
Circuit 8   page 94 of *Workouts for Women: Circuit Training*

Monday
Shoulders and Arms   page 18
Chest and Back   page 30

Tuesday
Lower Body   page 42
Abdominals and
   Lower Back   page 55

Wednesday
Shoulders and Arms   page 18
Abdominals and
   Lower Back   page 55

Thursday
Circuit 9   page 105 of *Workouts for Women: Circuit Training*

Friday
Rest Day

Saturday
Rest Day

5 Day Week 4

Sunday
Circuit 10   page 116 of *Workouts for Women: Circuit Training*

Monday
Lower Body   page 42
Chest and Back   page 30

Tuesday
Circuit 1   page 16 of *Workouts for Women: Circuit Training*

Wednesday
Shoulders and Arms   page 18
Abdominals and Lower Back   page 55

Thursday
Circuit 2   page 27 of *Workouts for Women: Circuit Training*

Friday
Rest Day

Saturday
Rest Day

CHAPTER 10
Creating a Workout

129

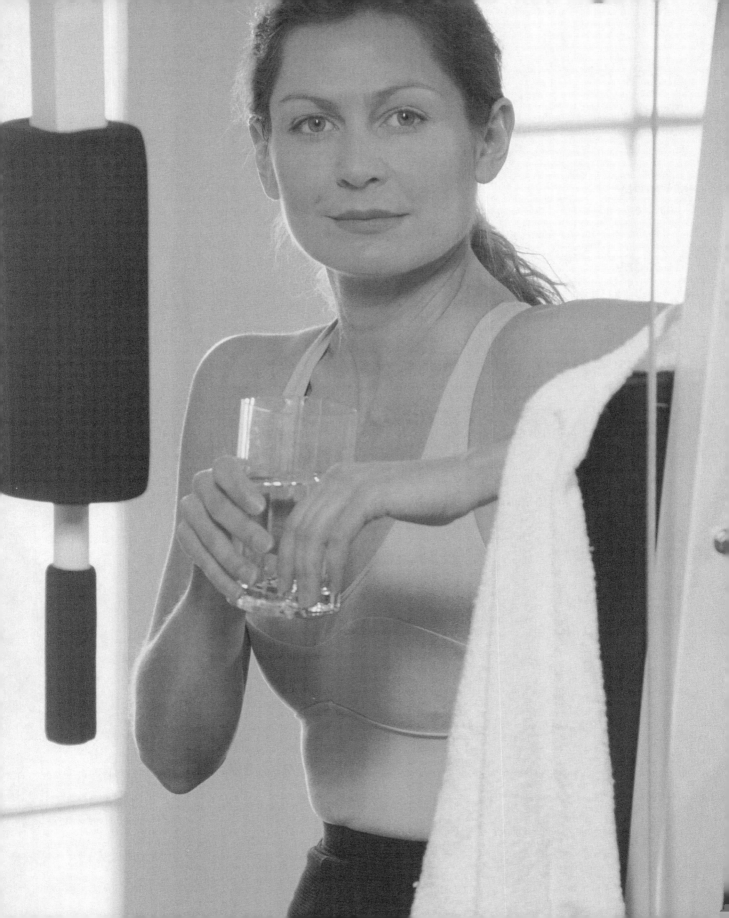

CHAPTER 11

Final Thoughts

Determination is defined as being resolute and unwavering in your direction. In order to succeed in life, you must have determination to overcome inevitable distractions, oppositions and obstacles. The five actions of determination are:

1. Setting personal and attainable goals

2. Ignoring distractions

3. Not giving in to discouragement

4. Facing challenges and changes head on

5. Not letting anything stop you

Determined individuals have vision. Without purpose, you have no fuel, no fire inside and little chance of reaching your goals. Be certain that you identify clear goals for yourself and then add in a dose of determination as you journey steadily toward meeting your goals.

You have the ability to lose weight, tone up, sculpt your body and experience the reality of being a strong, healthy woman. You deserve to be your best! Go ahead and make the commitment to begin today if you have not done so already. Empower yourself as a woman by making fitness a part of your lifestyle!

In fitness and in health,

Joni Hyde

Joni Hyde, Your Personal Trainer

Please visit me on the Web at www.WorkoutsforWomen.com, where you will find many free resources as well as other products to help you meet your fitness goals.

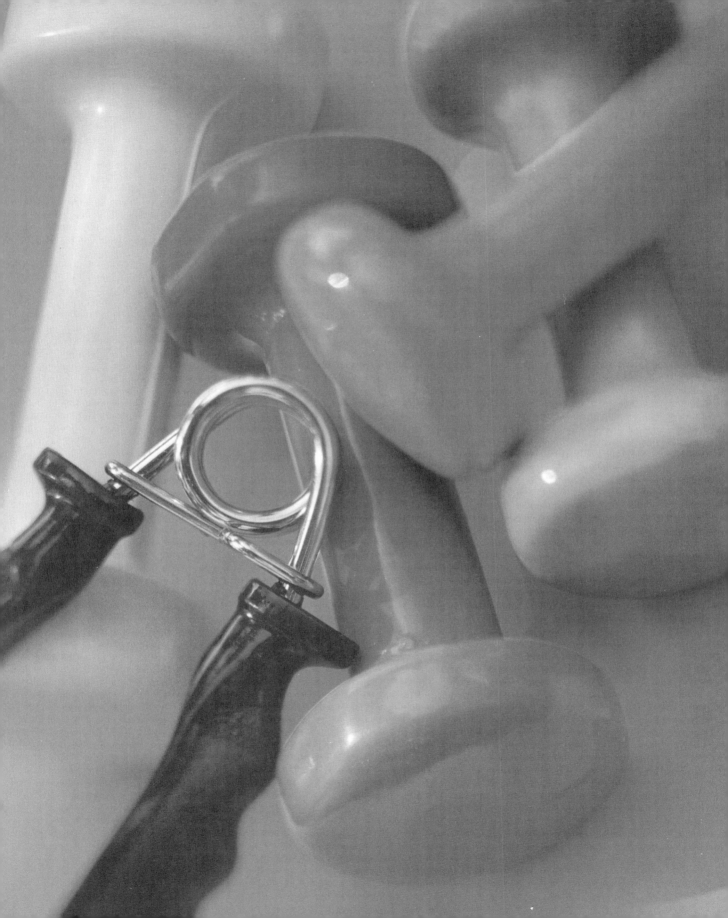

Workout Log

Instructions

Use this Workout Log to track your weekly workouts and keep you focused. Photocopy the weekly workout log as many times as you need.

For each day of the week, fill out what routine, circuit, or aerobics activity you followed, as in the sample workout log on page 134. You should also document the amount of weight you used for each Zone. Remember, as you progress, you should increase the weight you use to make the workout challenging, not impossible, to complete.

SAMPLE WORKOUT LOG

Start Date: **May 7th** End Date: **May 13th**

	EXERCISE NAME	WEIGHTS
SUNDAY	Shoulders and Arms Routine A	10
	Lower Body Routine B	15
MONDAY	REST	
TUESDAY	Chest and Back Routine A	10
	Abs and Lower Back Routine A	10
	30 minutes of cycling	
WEDNESDAY	REST	
THURSDAY	Total Body	10
	30 minutes of cycling	
FRIDAY	REST	
SATURDAY	REST	

WOR**K**OUT LOG

Work**o**uts for Women

WORKOUT LOG

Start Date: _____ End Date: _____

EXERCISE NAME	WEIGHTS
SUNDAY	
MONDAY	
TUESDAY	
WEDNESDAY	
THURSDAY	
FRIDAY	
SATURDAY	

APPENDIX A
Workout Log

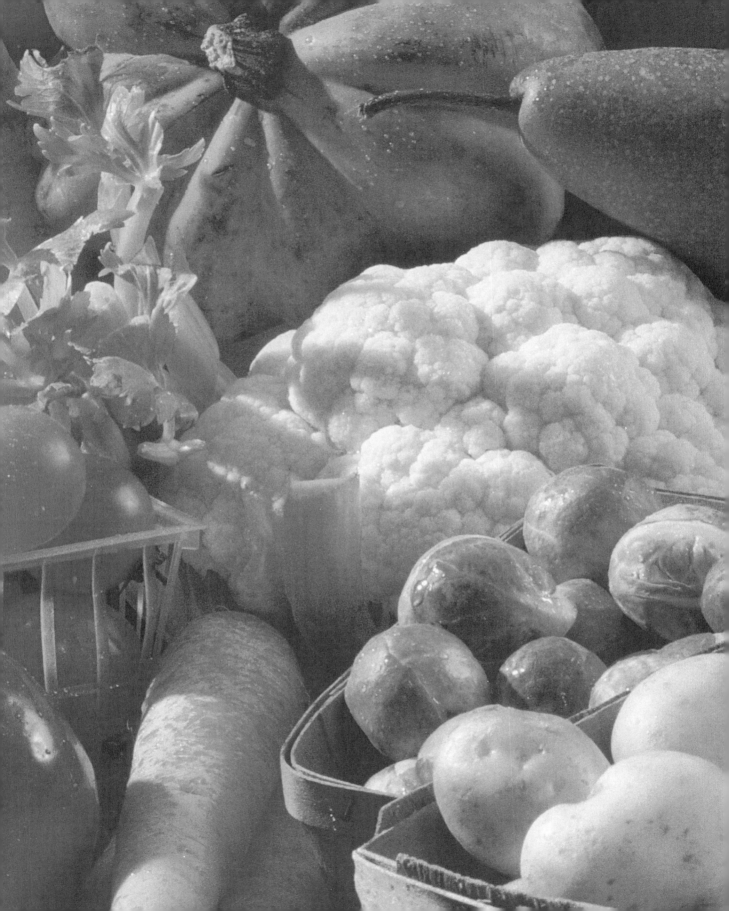

Food Journal

For optimal success, monitor your food consumption by keeping a visual record. Use the food journal to record the time you eat, what you eat and any activity that you were doing while you ate. It's also very helpful to track your mood at the time you were eating. This enables you to observe patterns in how activities and moods affect your food choices. Once you pinpoint what is negatively affecting your food choices you can work on making the appropriate changes.

For instance, perhaps you have a tendency to snack on crackers or cookies in the early evening while watching TV. With that knowledge, you can now plan to have a healthier alternative snack on hand for that time of the day since you know that is normally your prime snacking time. Another possible solution is to do something different during that time of the day to break the habit, such as taking a walk or reading a book in a different room instead of sitting where you normally do to snack.

SAMPLE FOOD JOURNAL

Day/Time	Food	Activity
3/25 7 am	Egg and cheese with bagel, hot tea	Breakfast watching news, relaxed
11 am	1/4 cup trail mix	Relaxed, working at desk
1 pm	Turkey and Swiss cheese wrap, grapes	Relaxed, at kitchen table
4 pm	1 cup bean soup, 4 whole-wheat crackers	A little nervous, thinking about job interview later this week
6:45 pm	Chicken cordon bleu and salad	Tired, long day
9:30 pm	Graham crackers ... too many!	Watching TV, bored, lonely
3/26 6 am	Cheerios and 1/2 cup yogurt	Breakfast watching news, relaxed
12:30 pm	Two Taco Bell burritos	Driving, rushing to meeting
8 pm	TV dinner and bowl of ice cream	Tired!
10 pm	Vanilla wafers and milk	Watching news, tired!
3/27 6 am	Fruit and yogurt	Relaxed, day off today
12:30 pm	Chicken caesar salad	Lunch out with friend, shopping day at the mall, relaxed
6:30 pm	Two slices cheese pizza	Food court with friend at the mall, tired
3/28 6 am	Yogurt and fruit	Nervous about interview tomorow
11 am	1/4 cup trail mix	Relaxed, eating at desk while working
1 pm	Tuna salad sandwich, grapes	Relaxed, lunch break
6:30 pm	Salmon and sweet potato, salad	Relaxed
9:30 pm	Graham crackers ... too many again.	Nervous about interview tomorow

FOOD JOURNAL

Workouts for Women

138

FOOD JOURNAL

Day/Time	Food	Activity

About The Author

Joni Hyde, a native of St. Petersburg, Florida, is dedicated to women's fitness. She is a Certified Personal Trainer through the American Council on Exercise, a Certified Health/Fitness Instructor through the American College of Sports Medicine, a Certified Aerobics and Fitness Instructor through the Aerobics and Fitness Association and a member of IDEA, Health and Fitness Association. With over 15 years of professional experience, Joni is well respected in the fitness community. She has worked with Tony Little, Body by Jake and Jeff Everson on various projects. In addition, she has made several television appearances, including a 4-week segment for an NBC affiliate in which she was the key expert on women's fitness. Joni's work has been featured in numerous publications, such as *Time, Self, Fitness, Shape, Consumer Reports on Health, Seventeen, Vive Magazine* and *Prevention.*

In 1998, Joni launched www.WorkoutsForWomen.com, an online complete training program, including personal encouragement and feedback plus support groups and life counselors. During her own pregnancy, the Web site was expanded to include a specially tailored fitness program for moms-to-be. In 2004, she produced the energetic and interactive Workouts for Women: Circuit Shaping DVD. Her first book, *Workouts For Women: Circuit Shaping* was published in January 2005 and Joni is excited to present this second book, *Workouts For Women: Weight Training.*

Looking toward the future, Joni's goal remains to establish empowerment in women through a lifestyle that embraces physical fitness. Joni, with the support of her husband David, continues to be a positive and healthy role model for women and especially for her 5-year-old daughter, Lindsey.

Visit us at www.WorkoutsforWomen.com for lots of free fitness information, articles, tips, and tools.

Special Book Buyers Discount Code: Book0206

Available for online purchases. Enter this discount code during checkout to receive 10% off your first purchase in our Fitness Store at www.WorkoutsforWomen.com

Workouts for Women: Circuit Shaping DVD or VHS
Bursting with over 90 different exercises, these 10 total-body circuit shaping routines can each be completed in less than 12 minutes. This is ideal if you are short on time or just getting back into exercise. For a longer and more challenging workout, simply choose complete 2, 3, or 4 circuits for up to a 45 minute workout.

Workouts for Women: Circuit Shaping Book
This book is the perfect companion guide to go along with the video! In *Workouts for Women : Circuit Shaping*, you'll learn how to circuit train at home or the gym and how to start burning fat in just 12 minutes a day.

Join the Online Personal Training "Achievers Club"
Don't go it alone! Receive guidance and support from the Leaders in Women's Fitness. Each week a new circuit training workout is available for you to view online. Stay on course with our online Accountability System. Tools to track your progress and more.

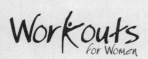